Pastoral counselling models for perinatal and postpartum episodes

Carl Davis

Published by Carl Davis, 2024.

While every precaution has been taken in the preparation of this book, the publisher assumes no responsibility for errors or omissions, or for damages resulting from the use of the information contained herein.

PASTORAL COUNSELLING MODELS FOR PERINATAL AND POSTPARTUM EPISODES

First edition. January 24, 2024.

ISBN: 979-8224344338

Written by Carl Davis.

Pastoral counselling models

for

Perinatal and

Postpartum episodes.

This Book is dedicated to all Mothers, especially my wife, Ronel and daughter-in-law, Chantell.

You know firsthand the emotional challenges of giving birth!

INTRODUCTION

Rubin's Stages of maternal psychological adaptation:

Reva Rubin postulates the following stages that a woman goes through after birth:

Taking in / dependent Phase

- First 3 days post partum.
- Focused on self, not infant, on her own needs for sleep & rest.
- Passive , dependent & can't make decisions.
- Need to discuss labour experiences.
- The sense of wonderment when looking at the neonate.

Taking Hold Phase:

- Last from the 3rd to 10th day postpartum.
- Focus on the infant.
- Active, independent & can make decisions.
- Initiates self-care activities, focus on bowels, bladder & breastfeeding.
- Responds to instruction about infant care & self-care.
- May express a lack of confidence in caring for the neonate.

Letting go:

- Last from 10 days to 6 weeks postpartum.
- The woman finally redefines her new role.
- See self as separate from the infant.
- Gives up fantasized image of her child and accepts the real

one.
- Readjustment.

What is Prenatal Depression?

Depression related to childbearing can occur during pregnancy is called "Prenatal **Depression**" or "**Antenatal Depression**"

Who is affected?

- According to the American College of Obstetricians and Gynecologists, about 10 percent of new mums experience postpartum depression —
- Up to 80% of new mothers cry easily or feel stressed following the birth of a baby. When this happens within the first two weeks following birth, it is called "baby blues."
- However, some women experience a deep sadness that doesn't go away or comes and goes. For other women, these feelings sometimes occur months after childbirth.

Reasons:

- Poor maternal care
- Family relationship problems
- Financial problems
- Abnormal levels of female hormones

Neurotransmitters and Depression:

Norepinephrine:

- Attention
- Motivation
- Pleasure
- Reward

Dopamine:

- Alertness
- Energy

Serotonin

- Obsessions and compulsions

Depletion of Norepinephrine, Dopamine and Serotonin leads to:

- Insomnia
- Anxiety
- Lethargy
- Loss of concentration
- Aggressive Behavior
- Attention deficit problem
- Sadness
- Suicidal thoughts

The Role of Hormones in Depression:

―――

Oestrogen

Oestrogen is the Female steroid hormone and makes a woman more susceptible to stress, anxiety and depression when its level is low.

PERINATAL DEPRESSION

Biological causes of perinatal depression

F luctuations in female reproductive hormones affect the neurochemical pathway which leads to prenatal depression.

Other functions of Progesterone besides maintaining the pregnancy is to regulate the female's mood, sleep, aggressive behaviour and anxiety

Effects of such depression:

- Mother: At high risk because of postpartum depression, premature labour, GIT problems, psychosis, deprived health conditions

- Fetus and child: Low birth weight, premature baby, cardiovascular problems, depression.

Feelings of Sadness:

- Caused by low levels of Oestrogen and Progesterone
- During pregnancy elevated levels of Corticotropin Releasing Hormone remains unbound which causes sadness (Florio et al., 2003).[1]
- Workload, joint family, being multiparous.

Loss of Interest:

Loss of pleasure and interest in daily activities during the period of pregnancy is due to tiredness and body aches (Gelder et al., 2005).[2]

Suicidal Thoughts:

Absent in most of the females, while some experienced mild and moderate feelings due to family problems and severe depression. The rate of suicide in gestational period is low

Crying:

Gestational Pre-eclampsia (gestational hypertension) occurs which can lead to crying and sadness during pregnancy

14

Irritation:

Irritation feeling during pregnancy is due to the decreased level of mood-regulating hormones oestrogen and progesterone (Macqueen et al., 2003).[3]

Social Avoidance:

Changes in a female's body make them feel that they don't look attractive in her own eyes and in other's eyes. Pregnant women who are depressed avoid social functions and social gatherings (Murray et al., 2003).[4]

Fatigue and Tiredness:

Fatigue in 1st trimester because a large amount of energy is required for building life support system. As females enter the second-trimester fatigue subsides (Campbell et al., 2004). Fatigue again starts in the third trimester because the fetus puts pressure and extra load on the body (Kiserud et al., 2004)[5]

Mood Swings:

Mood swings are mostly experienced during the first trimester and then again in the third trimester when the body prepares for birth (Peter et al., 2004).[6]

Mood changes during pregnancy are caused by physical stress, fatigue, metabolic changes, variation in hormones (such as oestrogen and progesterone) that has an effect on the brain and causes depression (Morrison et al., 2006)[7]

Appetite Changes:

The reason of loss of appetite during the third trimester is due to the increased level of progesterone which relaxes stomach & intestinal muscles that lead to Gastro oesophagal Reflux Disease (GERD) and ultimately loss of appetite (Niebyl et al., 2010)[8]

Anxiety due to weight gain:

Weight gain in pregnancy is related to fetal growth and this weight is attributed to additional blood volume, the weight of the uterus, placental weight, the weight of the fetus and extra fluid during the period of pregnancy (Feig et al., 1995).[9]

Body Pain:

Females reported a backache in the first and (most of the females reported) it in the third trimester. Backache and pelvic pain were reported most seeing that the fetus puts pressure on the lower back, abdominal muscles and pelvis.

Disturbances in sleeping cycles:

Sleep in gestational women is interrupted by fetal movements/physical discomfort and increases if a woman is depressed (Hiscock et al., 2001).[10]

This leads to poor sleep quality, decreased sleep efficiency and increased wakefulness, in the third trimester of pregnancy (Saletu et al., 2001)[11]

PERINATAL DEPRESSION IN FATHERS

While the phenomenon of depression during and following pregnancy in women is widely appreciated (and often associated with weight gain and/or antenatal weight retention), the effect of pregnancy on the mood of fathers is less appreciated.

- A recent study by James Paulson and Sharnail Bazemore from the Virginia Medical School, Norfolk, VA, just published in the Journal of the American Medical Association, throws new light on this interesting issue.[12]

- The researchers performed a meta-analysis of 43 studies that documented depression in fathers between the first trimester and the first postpartum year involving 28 004 participants.

- Although there was substantial heterogeneity between the rates of paternal depression between studies, the average rate of paternal depression in the antenatal period (during pregnancy) was about 10% but increased to about 25% during the 3 to 6-month postpartum period (after birth).

Findings:

- While paternal depression was more likely in the presence of maternal depression, this was by no means a strong predictor of paternal mood disorder.

- These findings have important implications.

- Not only is it important to also be wary of mood disorders in expecting and new fathers (especially if the mother has mood problems), but these mood disorders in fathers may need to be addressed.

Coping Fathers:

This is of particular importance given the emerging evidence that paternal depression may have substantial emotional, behavioural and developmental effects on the infant.

Furthermore, it may well be that paternal Prepartum depression could contribute to weight gain in dads.

Thus, prevention, screening and interventions for depression should likely be focused on the couple rather than on the individual parent.

POSTPARTUM EPISODES

Then, what is Postpartum disturbance?

Introduction

Highest vulnerability is in first 3 months after delivery

Three types of postpartum disturbances:

Postpartum blues ("baby blues")

Postpartum depression

Postpartum psychosis

Postpartum depression should be distinguished from postpartum adjustment

Many new mums feel happy one minute and sad the next. If you feel better after a week or so, you probably just had the "baby blues." If it takes you longer to feel better, you may have postpartum depression.[13]

Health professionals have told us that they become considerably involved with women they suspect of being depressed, but they are often unsure of what to do. With adequate training, support and liaison with other services, it should be possible to develop a structured and effective approach to promoting the psychological well-being of women during the postnatal period.

Historical development of Post-Partum Depression:

———

Much of the historical data on postpartum mood disorders is available from Europe. Although there existed a hospital for postpartum psychiatric diseases in France by 1858, women's issues were often minimized.

"Folie des nourrices" or psychosis of nursing was recognized but often only as a legitimate reason to get rid of a wife and have her sent to an asylum.

In 1926, a paper by Strecker and Ebaugh erroneously concluded that there was no psychosis designated as postpartum. It was not until the 4th edition of the DSM in 1994 that the postpartum onset of a psychiatric illness was used as a specifier.

"Baby Blues"

Postpartum or Maternity blues is the most frequently observed postpartum mood disturbance. Symptoms are generally transient and non-pathologic.

Maternity or "Baby" Blues Symptoms:

- Mood fluctuation, tearfulness, heightened reactivity
- Occurs within 3-5 days after delivery
- Appears unrelated to environmental stressors
- Not a psychiatric illness, but a frequently experienced physiological event for most new mothers
- No clinical intervention needed; usually resolves within 2 weeks of birth
- a mild, short-lived depression
- Anxiety
- Sadness
- Irritability
- Crying
- Headaches
- Exhaustion
- A sense of inadequacy

What is Post-Partum Depression?

- A more severe form of depression that can develop within the first six months after giving birth.
- Feelings such as sadness, anxiety and restlessness can be so strong that they interfere with daily tasks.
- Rarely, a more extreme form of depression known as postpartum psychosis can develop.

Although there is still no specific diagnosis of postpartum illness, the specifier allows for:

———

- A diagnosable illness that can be related to childbirth;
- A diagnostic code that allows the provider to be paid and pharmacy payments and follow up visits to be garnered.
- A categorization that will allow further research into these disorders.
- Feeling of being "out of control" during childbirth
- Have had depression or PND before
- Do not have a supportive partner
- Premature or sick baby
- Loss of own mother as a child
- Various stresses and anxieties
- Lack of, or too much, interest in the baby
- Poor self-care
- Loss of interest in otherwise normally stimulating activities
- Social withdrawal and isolation
- Poor concentration, confusion
- Exhaustion, fatigue
- Sluggishness
- Sleeping problems (not related to screaming baby)
- Appetite changes
- Headaches
- Chest pain
- Heart Palpitations
- Hyperventilation

R isk Factors:

- Self or family history of mental illness or substance abuse
- Marital or financial stresses
- Birth complications
- Lack of self-confidence as a parent
- Problem's with baby's health
- Major life changes around time of delivery
- Lack of support or help with baby
- The mother being of young age
- Severe premenstrual syndrome

What promotes Mental Wellbeing?

- It may be different things for every person
- Mental wellbeing will only be achieved if you have all your basic human needs met
- Maslow's Hierarchy of Needs is a good place to start searching for what gives us mental wellbeing
    - The need to give & receive attention (friends, family, social network)
    - Taking need of the mind-body connection (breath, sleep, food, exercise etc)
    - The need for purpose (goals, work, parents)
    - Connection to something bigger than oneself (religion, clubs, a cause/purpose)
    - The need for creativity & stimulation (learning new skills)
    - The need to feel understood & connected (intimacy, partnership)
    - The need to feel a sense of control

How do we normally deal with changes?

- Having a sense of control
- Sense of knowing/knowledge
- Confidence in your own ability (body/mind)
- Fear of unknown is removed
- Informed decisions
- Information gathered from others – history/research
- Tools and coping skills to help you with the process

Having a baby!

- If we feel the need to prepare for a 'normal challenge in life' why do we not prepare for labour, childbirth and parenting to the same degree?
- Antenatal classes give information on 'signs of labour', 'pain management' and 'medical intervention' but they fail to prepare us for the day of labour or parenting.
- Birth Secrets courses and hypnosis is a wonderful tool in preparing you for labour, birth and parenting.

LOSS: major issue in PPD (Nicholson)[14]

- Loss of Autonomy
- Loss of Time
- Loss of Appearance
- Loss of Femininity
- Loss of Sexuality
- Loss of Occupational identity

Loss of Autonomy & Time

- Autonomy—personal freedom
- The women feel that they just can't pick up and leave whenever they wish (vacation, hanging out with friends)
- They have to tend to the baby instead of just themselves
- Being a parent is a "24 hour, full-time job"
- In a case study done, several women were interviewed on this subject. One woman said that the "new baby's arrival eliminated time for her and her husband to be on their own together for at least 18 [more] years.

Loss of appearance:

- Anxiety about the loss of their former appearance
- Time plays into trying to keep up personal looks
- They don't feel comfortable with the changes in their bodies after having a baby
- They don't like the fact they can't wear the same clothes or the same type of clothes as they once did before being pregnant.

- Developed anxiety about their appearance—saw the changes as negative

Loss of femininity and Sexuality:

- Because of the anxiety about their appearance and the shape of their body after pregnancy they do not feel that their spouse would be attracted to them as much.
- Worried about body size/shape
- Self-image changed
- Had to think of themselves are more motherly beings than sexual beings

Loss of occupational identity:

The women have feelings of loss concerning:

- loss of power

- loss of opportunity
- loss of relationship w/ partners, friends
- loss of finances
- Debate whether or not to go back to work or to stay at home with the child
- Many have feelings of guilt

Dr Grantly Dick-Read and Fear-Tension-Pain Syndrome

- "Fear is the cause of tension within the body"
- Scientists discovered in mid-seventies that a source of natural analgesia was within the body
- Endorphins – neuropeptides in the brain and pituitary gland (80 times stronger than morphine)
- Endorphins produce a tranquil, amnesiac condition
- Adrenaline effects birth in a negative way
- Muscles tighten and blood supply is reduced in the uterus as it moves to the arms and legs gearing you for fight or flight response
- Adrenaline blocks the release of Endorphins (the body's natural painkillers)
- Endorphins – 80 times more effective than Morphine, you want those available during birth!
- Fear constricts muscles, not expands and dilates them!

The Uterus and relaxation:

- Increased blood supply/oxygen to Uterus through relaxation
- Muscles of Uterus are able to function effectively
- Each contraction works in harmony with your body and feels comfortable
- Each contraction is effectively dilating your cervix
- Relaxation aids in dilation of cervix
- Every 90 – 120 minutes

- Brain switches from left to right hemispheric dominance
- Breathing will change from left to right nostril dominance
- Bodies natural rest period

American Legislation:

The Post-Partum Depression Screening Legislation was enacted by the Senate and General Assembly and approved on April 13, 2006.[15]

The Law and Prenatal Period

Physicians, nurse midwives and other licensed health care professionals providing prenatal care to women shall provide:

- education to women and their families about postpartum depression in order to lower the likelihood that new mothers will continue to suffer from this illness in silence

Prior to discharge from the birthing facility:

All birthing facilities in the State shall:

- screen new mothers for PPD symptoms prior to discharge shall provide departing new mothers and fathers and other family members, as appropriate, with complete information about PPD, including its symptoms, methods of coping with the illness
and treatment resources

Patient & Family Education:

Physicians, nurse midwives and other licensed health care professionals providing prenatal and postnatal care to women shall:

- include fathers and other family members, as appropriate, in both the education and treatment processes to help them better understand the nature and causes of PPD

Postnatal Visits:

Physicians, nurse midwives and other licensed health care professionals providing postnatal care to women shall:

- screen new mothers for PPD symptoms prior:

- to discharge from the birthing facility
- at the first few postnatal check-up visits

Maternity Blues is not a psychiatric illness but a frequently experienced physiological event for most new mothers. It requires no clinical intervention and usually resolves within 2 weeks of birth. If present it does increase the risk of Postpartum Depression.

Adjustment Disorder defines a mother who is experiencing a greater than the normal adjustment that would be expected for a new mother. These women can benefit from short-term therapy focused on education, support, skills training and family interventions. The exact incidence is unclear as many women who experience this condition will not seek the clinical attention of any type.

The onset of Postpartum Depression according to DSM-IV is within four weeks. However clinical experience seems to indicate that the onset frequently occurs within 3 months but may present up to a year after the birth of the child. Many factors can contribute to the delay in the clinical identification of this disorder. Key factors may include denial of illness, shame and stigma, the intermittent and fluctuating course of the disorder.

Depression during the postpartum period affects 10% of patients and rises to about 20% in women who have experienced postpartum blues.

Untreated depression in the postpartum period is associated with health risks to the mother as well as the child in terms of cognitive, emotional, and social development.

Postpartum psychosis is rarely a condition that is considered a medical emergency when it develops. It typically has a dramatic onset and is categorized by psychotic symptoms, disorientation and disorganized behaviour.

The DSM-IV (Diagnostic and Statistical Manual of Mental Disorders, 4th Ed.) postpartum onset specifier for major depressive disorder is restricted to episodes with an onset within 4 weeks of delivery. However, some women develop symptoms more insidiously weeks or even months after childbirth.

Adjustment Disorder Symptoms:

- Development of emotional or behavioural symptoms, occurring within 3 months
- An identifiable stressor, the birth of a baby, causes a great deal of stress in the mother's life resulting in diminishing her coping mechanisms
- Psychotherapy is the treatment of choice for adjustment disorder, as it is seen as a normal reaction to a situational event[16]

As compared to Baby Blues, Adjustment disorder is pervasive.

Risk Factors for Post-Partum Depression:

- Prenatal depression/history of depression
- Prenatal anxiety/history of anxiety
- Experiencing stress in life
- Teen pregnancy
- Marital satisfaction / relationship
- Socioeconomic factors
- Obstetrical complications
- Among high and moderate risk factors for postpartum mood disorders most notable is any history of psychiatric illness, before or during the pregnancy.
- Anxiety, including panic attacks, obsessive-compulsive symptoms and general fearfulness very frequently accompany or are markers of depressive episodes.
- Substance abuse is a red flag for other co-morbid conditions, which the patient may be "self-medicating."
- The other most significant risk conditions concern lack of social support systems, which include the family of origin and marital relationship, and finally severe life stresses occurring during pregnancy.
- Although, less predictive as a risk factor is lower socioeconomic status.

Poverty and Depressed Mothers:

- 11% of infants living in poverty have Mum suffering from depression
- Mums can also be struggling with DV, substance abuse, and report fair health
- Mums breastfeed for shorter periods
- Although treatable depressed Mums do not receive care
- Depressed Mums in poverty already connected to services; therefore opportunity to identify depression and help seek treatment[17]

Social Isolation, Contributing Factors:

- Woman perceives herself as not supported; has low self-esteem
- Family lives at a distance, physically unavailable or culturally in conflict
- Cut off from friends
- Relationship discord, including emotional or physical abuse; desertion of spouse or significant other
- History of childhood sexual abuse

The perception of being not supported can be a central issue in a depressed post-partum mother, even if the facts do not support her perception.

In the case where multiple generations of relatively recent immigrants are living in a community, the extent of acculturation across generations may pose conflicts to the new mother who wishes either to reject or restrict cultural practices related to pregnancy and new motherhood. Ex: types of foods, the level of activity etc.

In our increasingly mobile society, new mothers may find themselves far away from family and friends and the isolating aspects of pregnancy have not given sufficient opportunity to create new friendships. When geographic or social circumstances already isolate a mother her relationship with her partner becomes even more important. If difficulties are present, the isolation can be profound.

Very young or older mothers may find themselves in the position of lacking social support or identification with others in their age group. For example, an adolescent mother may feel more isolated and resentful as her friends continue to enjoy their youth and freedom without such responsibilities. An older mother may find she has little in common with mothers in their twenties and early thirties because her birth story and life circumstances are different, while women her age may have already passed through the motherhood experience.

Within an isolated environment, the ability to put one's mood and feelings into proper context or perspective is difficult. Feelings of being totally cut off from the world and fear that depressive feelings will be harshly judged can prevent a new mother from seeking appropriate support.

Most important, perhaps, is the esteem in which a woman holds herself. Self-esteem and sexuality may be severely damaged by abuse, especially sexual abuse, which must be inquired about, as shame and pain may hinder spontaneous revelation.

Non-contributing Risk Factors to Postpartum Depression:

- Maternal Age
- Level of Education
- Number of Children
- Length of relationship with partner
- Gender of the child

- Feeling tired after delivery, broken sleep patterns, and not enough rest often keeps a new mother from regaining her full strength for weeks.
- Feeling overwhelmed with a new, or another, baby to take care of and doubting your ability to be a good mother.
- Feeling stress from changes in work and home routines. Sometimes, women think they have to be "super mum" or perfect, which is not realistic and can add stress.
- Having feelings of loss — loss of identity of who you are, or were, before having the baby, loss of control, loss of your pre-pregnancy figure, and feeling less attractive.
- Having less free time and less control over time.
- Having to stay home indoors for longer periods of time and having less time to spend with your partner and loved ones.

Obstetrical Risks:

These include complications during pregnancy, more than normal antenatal visits or lack of prenatal care, multiple prior terminations and multiple births in assisted pregnancies. In addition, hyperemesis and antenatal depression have also been identified as risk factors.

- Complications during the present pregnancy
- Frequent visits to the antenatal clinic
- Lack of prenatal care
- Increased number of sick days
- History of 2 or more elective terminations
- Delivery by cesarian section
- Hyperemesis
- Preterm labour (not delivery)
- Depression in antenatal period
- During pregnancy, the amount of two female hormones, oestrogen and progesterone, in a woman's body increases

greatly.

- In the first 24 hours after childbirth, the amount of these hormones rapidly drops back down to their normal non-pregnant levels.
- Researchers think the fast change in hormone levels may lead to depression, just as smaller changes in hormones can affect a woman's moods before she gets her menstrual period.

Potential Effects of Postpartum Mood Disorders

When examining the potential effects of postpartum mood disorders, we can identify three areas of concern:

- Effects on The Mother/Infant Relationship
- Effects on Child Development
- Effects on the Partner Relationship

Postpartum depression can have an adverse effect on maternal-infant interactions.

Research also shows that postpartum depression has a small but significant effect on children's cognitive and emotional development. (Beck, CT, 1998).[18] The effect of PPD on cognitive development, such as language and IQ have been documented particularly among boys. (Grace SL, et al 2003).[19]

Lastly, several aspects of child outcome have been found to be associated with postpartum depression. This includes the child's behaviour with the mother, behavioural disturbance at home, and the content and social patterns of play at school. (Murray L, et al 1999)[20]

- Negative Mother/Infant Relationship
- Delayed Child Development
- Altered Partner Relationship

Long-term Effects of Maternal Depression on Children

- Longitudinal study of 5,000 mother/child pairs
- Severity and chronicity of maternal depression related to child behaviour problems and lower vocabulary scores at age 5[21]

How Depression Can Influence Breastfeeding:

Most mothers are told that "breast is best" from many respected professional sources. Mothers are encouraged to breastfeed their baby for up to one year.

While the public health message about breastfeeding is good news for the baby and reasonable for a healthy mother, it can feel like another pressure for a mother who is trying to cope with a mood disorder. Depression can make it difficult to read the baby's cues and to successfully navigate the ongoing efforts that surround breastfeeding. Mothers with Postpartum Mood Disorders may require additional education, support and information regarding breastfeeding. One might consider recommending a lactation consultant or a postpartum doula to facilitate the breastfeeding experience if the mother chooses to nurse.

Maternal Depression Still-Face Paradigm:

Watch how a baby may react to mother's changing facial expressions. Pay special attention to the child's facial expressions and movements in this example. Please be aware that the mother was instructed on how to change her interaction with the baby during this clip, from being playful to having a flat affect, back to playful. After the clip, we will explain the theories behind the study in which this pair was participating. Ask group for their observations and encourage brief discussion)

The Face-to-Face/Still-Face Paradigm (Cohn & Tronick, 1983[22]; Tronick and Field, 1986[23]) investigates the parent-child relationship with a focus on the infant's behavioural, affective and physiologic reactions during structured face-to-face infant-caregiver interactions. Studies have used the still-face paradigm to analyze split-screen videotaped episodes with both depressed and non-depressed mothers and their infants and toddlers. During the still-face episodes, the mothers are asked

1) to engage with infant spontaneously,

2) to turn away from infant and the return with a simulated depressive affect or still-face, and

3) to turn away again and, after a brief pause, to reunite and re-engage the infant in spontaneous affective interaction.

The affect and behaviour of depressed mothers have been shown to disrupt the infant's sense of control, emotional displays of joy and pleasure, and felt security in the relationship. The studies dramatize the complexity of infants effective responses with their mothers during the still-face and subsequent resparatory interactions during the reunion. During the still-face, infants of non-depressed mothers protest, gaze avert and may make efforts to regain the positive interaction with their mother. During the reunion, infants may show a mixed emotional reaction before fully re-engaging with a parent. The behaviour and affect of infants of depressed mothers seem to more closely mirror the effect of their mothers during each episode, with less of a range in effective responses.

The theory behind the research was not so much that a parent with a flat affect was distressing to a child—I think this could probably be proven fairly easily. The hypothesis was that a child who was routinely exposed to an effectually-flat parent would display markedly different interactions than a child that wasn't. The "control" dyad would show distress during the still-face, try to find ways to get a response from the mother, etc, which we saw in the video clip. The "experimental" dyad, however, would, in theory, show us a child who would have less distress during the still-face. Just as important, however, would be to see what types of differences were seen during the "normal play" portion of the interaction.

A structured clinical research paradigm such as the still-face is useful for identifying patterns that assist in understanding parent-child interactions. Used thoughtfully, these data and findings can contribute to our understanding of infant-parent relationships and lend guidance to sensitive and accurate naturalistic observations of infants and caregivers.

As you can see from the clip, infants of depressed mothers show Less effort to engage mother, more fussing and emotional dysregulation (which is the inability to calm oneself), difficulty regulating emotions and repairing/restoring interactions after a disruption.

Depressed mothers are less sensitively attuned and more behave in a more negative fashion towards infants than non-depressed mothers

Patterns of maternal behaviour with infants include 2 types:

- Intrusive: handling baby roughly, actively interfering and interrupting infant's activities, overt anger
- Withdrawn: Disengaged, unresponsive, effectively flat, not noting or supportive of infants activities

Depression in mother distressing to infant:

- Infant's subsequent distress contributes to severity of mother's depression as she feels she cannot comfort infant
- Infant's unresponsiveness also validates mothers' depressive sense of her parenting capacities and her experience of herself in relationships
- Mother's depressed mood & unpredictability leads to distress for infant that in turn impairs infant responsivity and

contingent responding
- Negative perceptions and fantasies "Ghosts in the Nursery"
- Impaired ability to consider the world from baby's point of view

PPD Screening:

———

The policies and recommendations from the postpartum mood disorders working group were incorporated into the legislation. The institution of screening for postpartum mood disorders was one of the four recommendations suggested as a standard of care both pre- and postnatally.

Blood tests can help your doctor determine whether an underactive thyroid is contributing to your signs and symptoms.

PPD Screening Tool

- A reliable and validated screening tool, such as the Edinburgh Postnatal Depression Scale (EPDS), or another appropriate test that assists in identifying warning signs for postpartum conditions.
- Screening is designed to assist, not replace, clinical judgment. Women should be further assessed before deciding on treatment.
- Consider additional mitigating factors, such as environmental and family issues, when considering patient risk levels.
- Document screening results & risk status on the medical record.
- Women should initially be screened at the 28-week prenatal office visit
- Give a copy of the results of the screening to the mother.
- Provide counselling regarding the implications of their risk status to the mother along with other family members as appropriate.
- Distribute educational, self-care and local resource materials.

- Encouraging participation in further evaluation for diagnosis and, if necessary, treatment from an appropriate primary care or mental health provider.
- Supplying referral information for services clinically appropriate up to and including emergency intervention.

Screening Tools:

- Postpartum Depression Predictors Inventory – Cheryl Beck
- Postpartum Depression Screening Scale – also Cheryl Beck – Self-administered followed by a clinician interview, copyright issues, reliability studied have been done but are not yet published
- Ante Partum Questionnaire – self-report, not widely used
- Zung Self-Rating Depression Scale – 20 item, self-report
- (Aaron) Beck Depression Inventory – not specifically for PPD, used in psychiatry, cost associated
- Other common screening tools with evidence of validity in the puerperium: Postpartum Depression Screening Scale (PDSS)[24]- 35-item Likert-type response scale consisting of 7 domains: sleeping/eating disturbances, anxiety/insecurity, emotional lability, cognitive impairment, loss of self, guilt/ shame, and contemplating harming oneself) and the 9-item Physician's Health Questionnaire (PHQ-9) [25]- PHQ-9 is the depression module, which scores each of the nine DSM-IV criteria as "0" (not at all) to "3" (nearly every day). It has been validated for use in primary care. It is not a screening tool for depression but it is used to monitor the severity of depression and response to treatment. However, it can be used to make a tentative diagnosis of depression in at-risk populations).
- The Antepartum Questionnaire (APQ) was developed in

1997 and evaluates in 24 questions the past and present time feelings of the puerperal on a number of subjects. A scoring of $\geq$ 46 should be considered for psychiatric evaluation and followed closely during the postpartum to detect possible signs of PPD.

- Edinburgh Postnatal Depression Scale (EPDS)

Edinburgh Postnatal Depression Scale:

The Edinburgh Postnatal Depression Scale[26] has been developed to assist primary care health professionals to detect mothers suffering from postnatal depression; a distressing disorder more prolonged than the "blues" (which occur in the first week after delivery) but less severe than puerperal psychosis. Previous studies have shown that postnatal depression affects at least 10% of women and that many depressed mothers remain untreated. These mothers may cope with their baby and with household tasks, but their enjoyment of life is seriously affected and it is possible that there are long-term effects on the family. The EPDS was developed at health centres in Livingston and Edinburgh. It consists of ten short statements. The mother underlines which of the four possible responses is closest to how she has been feeling during the past week.

Most mothers complete the scale without difficulty in less than 5 minutes. The validation study showed that mothers who scored above threshold 92.3% were likely to be suffering from a depressive illness of varying severity. Nevertheless, the EPDS score should not override clinical judgment. A careful clinical assessment should be carried out to confirm the diagnosis. The scale indicates how the mother has felt during the previous week and in doubtful cases, it may be usefully repeated after 2 weeks. The scale will not detect mothers with anxiety neuroses, phobias or personality disorder.

Instructions:

- The mother is asked to underline the response that comes closest to how she has been feeling in the previous 7 days.
- All ten items must be completed.
- Care should be taken to avoid the possibility of the mother discussing her answers with others.
- The mother should complete the scale herself unless she has limited English or has difficulty with reading.

This is not a diagnostic tool, but rather a screening tool. Refer the patient should a score of more than 1 be identified.

A positive answer to question 10 on the Edinburgh means that the woman is at risk for PPD. Implications of the score on question 10, self-harm. Health professionals without mental health qualifications who administer the scale often worry about positive scores on item 10 of the EPDS.

The majority of women with a small infant are unlikely to act on suicidal feelings.

There is little published evidence linking suicidal ideation and risk with response to item 10 on the EPDS. However, there is a strong correlation regarding thoughts of self-harm and might be more difficult for a health professional to recognize.

A positive score on item 10[27] should be taken seriously and action should be taken immediately. If the mother answers positively to question 10, you need to assess the severity of the situation and ask the following questions:

- Severity
- How often and how severe is the feeling?

- Has she made any previous attempts to harm herself or her baby?
- What is she looking forward to? Does she have a good support system who can help her see the positive factors in her life?
- Plan - Has she thought about how she will go about it? (Does she have a plan?)
- Has she got the means? (And are these likely to be effective?)
- Support System - What support does she have at home?
- If she has a partner, has she told him how she is feeling? Can she count on him to understand and give her emotional support? If she hasn't told him, would she like someone at the office or her doctor to help her to explain how she is feeling? If she doesn't have a partner or feels that she really can't tell him, is there anyone else who would be understanding (and not judgmental) and whose support she could realistically call on? Has she told this person or anyone else about her feelings? Could she phone this person and would they come if she feels bad?
- Do her parents know? (Is she close to them?)
- The questions should be asked in a supportive way encouraging the mother to tell her own story in her way.
- If the mother has a plan to hurt herself or the baby or is unable to answer questions satisfactorily she must not be left alone and should be accompanied to the nearest ER or Mental Health practitioner's office.

False Negatives Despite Screening

Inaccurate self-report

- Undiagnosed mood disorders
- Denial of illness

Fear of involvement of child protection agencies

Ability to mask symptoms especially if highly functional

Motherhood myth

Cultural Considerations

- Cultural learning- explore & understand the health beliefs, perceptions, practices, & preferences of the patient's culture
- Cultural competence -incorporate patient's preferences & practices, and respect patient's beliefs, values & perceptions
- Don't stereotype a culture
- Don't assume from a person's name or appearance that they belong to / practice a certain culture/religion
- Acculturation (cultural relativism): acquiring the norms, values, ideas, & behaviours of the dominant society
- Enculturation (ethnocentric): individuals retaining identification with their traditional ethnic group
- Culture impacts

- How a woman experience/ describe the experience of PMD
- How she copes with the illness
- How much stress she experiences
- Her willingness to seek care, adopt treatment or follow-up

We often see young women who have had lifelong mood disorders who come into treatment because those mood disorders have become unmanageable usually because of increased stressors. These women have been functional, even highly competent throughout their life. Self-report instruments can yield inaccurate results when masking symptoms have become a part of their overall functioning. Such patients can slip through the cracks. When administering a self-report, it may be prudent to have a staff member conduct the interview or review the findings with the person, as some encouragement may be needed to express a level of discomfort that a person has either learned to live with or is hesitant to admit.

In addition, if a pregnant woman has had previous experience postpartum illness necessitating the involvement of community agencies, she may be loath to repeat that experience for fear she may have her case reopened, lose the baby or have other children taken away, Such a woman may not be forthcoming in self-report or at interview.

Lastly, we are all familiar with the motherhood myth that joyous expectation should be the prevailing mood. This discrepant assumption can isolate a woman who is not feeling this maternal joy and make her unwilling or unavailable to disclose her symptoms of depression.

Complications:

- Left untreated, postpartum depression can last for up to a year or longer — taking a toll on the entire family.
- Untreated postpartum depression can interfere with mother-child bonding and cause family distress.
- Children of mothers with untreated postpartum depression are more likely to have behavioural problems, including sleeping and eating difficulties, temper tantrums and hyperactivity.
- Delays in language development are common as well.

Severe presentations and treatment:

- Antidepressants are a proven treatment for postpartum depression.
- If you're breastfeeding, it's important to know that any medication you take will enter your breast milk.

- Some antidepressants can be used during breastfeeding with little risk to your baby.
- But several antidepressants raise concerns for the baby, and various others have not been adequately tested to fully assess the risk.
- Work with your doctor to weigh the potential risks and benefits as you choose the treatment that's right for you.

Hormone Therapy:

Oestrogen replacement may help counteract the rapid drop in oestrogen that accompanies childbirth. However, oestrogen therapy after childbirth may decrease milk production and increase the risk of developing blood clots in the leg or lungs. As with antidepressants, weigh the potential risks and benefits of hormone therapy with a doctor.

Self-help:

- Make healthy lifestyle choices. Rest as much as you can. Exercise regularly. Try daily walks with your baby. Eat healthy foods — plenty of fruits, vegetables and whole grains. Avoid alcohol.
- Set realistic expectations. Don't pressure yourself to do everything. Scale back your expectations for the perfect household. Do what you can and leave the rest. Ask for help when you need it.
- Make time for yourself. If you feel like the world is coming down around you, take some time for yourself. Get dressed, leave the house and visit a friend or run an errand. Or schedule some time alone with your partner.
- Avoid isolation. Talk with your partner, family and friends about how you're feeling. Ask other mothers about their experiences. Ask your doctor about local support groups for new mums or women with postpartum depression.

Fathers and Postpartum Depression

Fathers can also develop a form of PPD because they also have to adjust to a new lifestyle with the addition of a new baby into the family.

They are affected by the emotional state of the mother and also have an added responsibility to care for the child while the mother is suffering.

- Lifestyle change
- Role of partner and child
- Sharing attention can lead to Drug & Alcohol use,
- social behaviour and increased risk taking,
- and sexually deviant behaviour
- Stress at work (working longer hours) b/c wife is on maternity leave
- Feeling physically separated
- Emotional attachment during and after pregnancy
- Planned or unplanned pregnancy
- 10% of American fathers had symptoms of depression

The child of a parent with PPD

An infant of a PPD mother can have:

- irregular sleep,
- more depressed affect,
- higher norepinephrine levels,
- and a lower vagal tone (which indicates that the infant is undergoing stress)
- and the body is reacting by releasing norepinephrine and the heart rate actually is slower in order for the body to deal with stressful activities—heart rate decreases and sympathetic activity increases.
- When toddlers these children are associated with having delays in verbal skills, having behaviour problems, and the school-readiness skills lack.
- When the children get older they tend to develop some behavioural/emotional problems—this puts them at a higher risk of developing depression themselves.
- It is suggested that child's social and learning ability and cognition will be affected
- Fathers with depression is thought to increase the likelihood that his children will act out or behave destructively
- Mothers with depression is associated with decreased overall health and learning problems with a greater risk of depression

Postpartum Psychosis or Mania
Common Symptoms:

Psychosis

Delusions

- Hallucinations

- Disorganized speech

- Disorganized behavior

- Symptoms are typically related to the infant, often with a religious flavour

- Marked changes of moods

Mania

Euphoria

- Decreased need for sleep

- More talkative

- Racing thoughts

- Distractibility

- Increased involvement in activities

- Excessive involvement in pleasurable but risky activities

Postpartum psychosis is a life-threatening psychiatric emergency that occurs in 0.1% of postpartum women often without significant premorbid symptoms.

Cognitive impairment

Thoughts of suicide and infanticide (hospital admission)

Women with bipolar affective disorder are at high risk. Up to 50% of those with bipolar disorder relapse in the early postpartum period often with psychotic symptoms.

Most patients with a postpartum psychosis have no previous history of psychiatric disorder.

Women with postpartum psychosis are at higher risk of AITD but also of clinical thyroid failure.

These data implicate thyroid dysfunction as an important clinical outcome in patients with postpartum psychosis.

AITD represents a potentially strong etiologic factor for the development of postpartum psychosis.

Screening for TPO antibodies is warranted in patients with postpartum psychosis.

Causes and Risk:

- lack of social and emotional support;
- a low sense of self-esteem due to a woman's postpartum appearance;
- feeling inadequate as a mother;
- feeling isolated and alone;
- having financial problems;
- and undergoing a major life change such as moving or starting a new job.

THE ONSET OF INTERVENTIONS:

All Christians who are actively involved in the battle between Light and Darkness will be in need of counselling some or other time. There are no real battles going on without casualties. Only those who are cowardly hiding while others are fiercely involved in the battle will come through unwounded. It is those soldiers who are a danger to the enemy that are often wounded severely because Satan is a strategist and he targets those who are a real danger to him and the advancement of his dark kingdom. Therefore Christians who are active in the battle often need restoration through counselling. Proper counselling is the work of those who had been restored themselves through the grace of God. Only those who have experienced the grace of restoration are fit to guide others because true Christian counselling is the sharing of experience and the discovery of truths rather than the teaching and application of techniques.

Christian counselling is based on the fact that no person will be fit to counsel others if he or she did not "take the medicine" and became healed by it. It is only after walking the minefield oneself that a person qualifies to guide others through their personal minefields or struggles. Any person becoming involved in counselling others must understand the fact that it is his or her own brokenness that qualifies him or her to be a Christian Counsellor. This fact is clearly stated in Gal 6:2-3: Help carry one another burdens, and in this way, you will obey the law of Christ. If you think you are something when you really are nothing, you are only deceiving yourself.

There is a big difference between Christian counselling and Psychological assistance or therapy. One must be sure that the person being counselled is indeed a brother or sister in Christ. Those who did not accept Christ as personal Saviour cannot be counselled on a Christian basis and such people must first accept Christ as Saviour at the onset of the counselling process, or understand that they will be guided during the counselling process to make a choice for Christ. This absolute decision will determine the outcome of the whole counselling process. It serves no purpose to waste valuable time on non-Christians because the only real solution that can be offered to any person is a solution based on the reality of Christ and His involvement through the Holy Spirit in our lives. Should one discover that the person coming for help finds it difficult to accept Christ; such person must be referred or advised to seek help from psychologists or other human support organisations. One must, however, guard against being critical or harsh towards any person in need because people in need often experience a darkness of the soul in which even God becomes absent. It is, therefore, wise to give total acceptance and first guide the person towards understanding your own brokenness, doubts, failures and humanness as a believer who is only allowed to act as a counsellor by the grace of God.

Why Counselling?

In your ministry as a pastor or spiritual leader of a group of Christians, it will often happen that you will encounter individual believers (or non-believers) in a one-on-one situation. Although it often seems more comfortable, if not downright easier, to deal with people from the relatively safe position of the pulpit, or as a facilitator in a small group, those are definitely not the only ways to proclaim the Word of God, to teach people, or to address certain specific issues.

Very often you will find your ministry to be most effective when dealing with people on an individual basis. There is much greater opportunity for deep fellowship and true personal contact. There is also often greater personal honesty between pastor and believer because there are no other people around whose presence might otherwise be quite intimidating.

The problem for many pastors, however, is that they often have no clear sense of exactly what they are doing or are supposed to be doing in such a counselling situation. What are the rules of the game? What is the objective? Is there a common objective in dealing with the many kinds of problems one could encounter in one's ministry? Should all problems be dealt with in the same way? Is there a recipe for success?

These could at first glance appear to be rather daunting questions, and in a sense they are, because the pastor always has to remain pastor in the complete sense of the word: a servant of God, not speaking with his own voice or ideas, but with the voice of God's Word, presenting God's love, God's grace, God's demands...

However, in this sense, his position is no different from that in the pulpit or the small group, and this also makes it a lot easier. Exactly because the pastor is a servant of God and not acting in his personal capacity, he is not left to his own devices!

The Word of God is as much a guide to the pastor himself in doing the work he has been called for, as it is a guide to be presented and explained to the faithful. Moreover, it is an authoritative guide and must be followed. It does not merely present good guidelines which can be tried out and rejected if they turn out to be impractical!

In these first lectures, therefore, we have to search the Word of God for his teaching regarding the task of the pastor counselling the individual believer.

In order to do this, we will focus on two important issues:

The meaning of life:

Everything we do, think, say and desire is influenced by our view regarding the meaning of life. When we say, for instance, that life is all about being happy, everything we do will be devoted to making us as happy as possible.

If you know someone's beliefs about the meaning of life, his actions will also make sense to you, because you will have a clear understanding of his motives. On the other hand, if you yourself have a clear understanding of what the meaning of life should be according to Scripture, it will not be so difficult to offer guidance on correct patterns of thought or behaviour.

It will be explained at a later stage that one of your prime objectives in counselling is to bring believers' lives into conformity to God's plan for them - and this is what the true meaning of life is all about!

The basic framework of the believer's life:

———

Many believers have no clear understanding of the basic course their lives will take precisely because they are believers. Having a clear grasp of this course will help both you and the people you counsel to make sense of individual experiences and problems, and also to seek solutions to problems in such a way that the overall design of their lives is served.

We will describe this course of life as the journey from justification through sanctification to glorification.

The Meaning of Life?

People offer many different answers to the question: "What is the meaning of life?". Some answer: the enjoyment of all good things in life. Others might say: to be happy. There will be those who say: to make money. There will be others who say: to have children. And so it continues: to have power and to rule; to govern the universe; to be successful; to reach ultimate self-actualization and self-expression; to have peace; to create harmony in a dissonant world.

On the more negative side, some people might give the following answers: man lives for the pleasure of a cruel god, or to serve demanding forefathers. Some might even go to the extreme of saying that man only lives in order to die, and that life, therefore, has no meaning at all!

The answer anyone gives when asked as to the meaning of life will ultimately depend on his or her experience of life in a world which is not always the most wonderful place to be. However, our experience can never be the ultimate source of truth. What do we learn from the Bible about the reason for man's existence?

Man in Paradise

In Genesis 1 the story of the creation of the world is told. It is very well known to almost all people who have ever read the Bible. In it, we read how God created the world in six days and rested on the seventh.

During the first five days, God started to shape and fill the formless and empty mass of the earth: He created light; water under and above the expanse; dry ground and vegetation; the sun, moon and stars; all the animals of the world. Then, when everything was in place, He created once more: mankind!

Then God said, "Let us make man in our image, in our likeness, and let them rule over the fish of the sea and the birds of the air, over the livestock, over all the earth, and over all the creatures that move along the ground."

So God created man in his own image, in the image of God he created him; male and female he created them. God blessed them and said to them, "Be fruitful and increase in number; fill the earth and subdue it. Rule over the fish of the sea and the birds of the air and over every living creature that moves on the ground."

(Genesis 1:26-28).

Mankind was created to be the image of God, to fill the earth, to subdue it and to rule over it.

In Genesis 2 we also read how God placed man in his garden to work it and to take care of it (Genesis 2:15).

What does it mean for man to be "created in the image of God"? It means:

- That every human being is worthy of honour and respect. Even after the fall, it is still given as the reason why no man should kill (Genesis 9:6) or curse (James 3:9) another man;

- That man originally resembled God in righteousness and holiness (Ephesians 4:24), as well as knowledge (Colossians 3:10);

- That man reflects the glory of God like a mirror, thus making God "visible" within his creation (2 Corinthians 3:18);

- That man is God's representative or ambassador, ruling in his name, dealing with creation as God would;

- That man is also God's servant, responsible first of all to God, with the express task of cultivating God's world and generally taking care of it (this includes all fellow human beings);

- That man is able to communicate with God because he is the same kind as God (although the radical distinction between man and God should never be forgotten!).

What, then, was the reason for man's existence when he was first created? It is clear from Genesis 1:26-28 that man was created first of all for fellowship with God (in prayer and worship), and for serving God (in worship and in taking care of creation and his fellow man - compare Matthew 25:31-46).

This is affirmed by the author of the letter to the Hebrews, in Hebrews 13:15-16, when he ascribes two functions to the believer as a priest in the service of God:

- to make an offering of praise to God and

- to do good to others and share with them.

This corresponds to entering into a deeper relationship with God and more effectively pleasing him through worship and service - which should also be the deepest motivation for solving any personal problem.

Fellowship with God, worship of God and representational service in this world are the three components of what we may call: the glorification of God. Man exists only to glorify God! Not his own well-being, nor that of other people, but God's glory is the primary reason for man's existence.

Man after Paradise

When Adam and Eve first sinned, they rebelled against the very reason for their existence: they no longer wanted to serve and glorify God, but only to serve and glorify themselves. From that day on, all people have worked and lived with only one purpose in mind - to be regarded with respect by others.

People devote their lives to doing good, to becoming rich, to having big families, to achieving maximum success, to gaining absolute power - all for the sake of regaining a sense of being worth at least something, a sense of being accepted by others.

Almost all suffering in this world, all wars, all injustice, all perversity can eventually be traced to this root cause: the search for being accepted and respected by others as being someone significant and meaningful.

You will also witness this in your ministry in this broken world. Husbands will blindly destroy their marriages, because not their wives, but they themselves with all their insecurities and needs, will be in the centre of their lives. They will love themselves rather than their wives.

The same can be said of the relation between parents and children, between brothers and sisters, between friends, between fellow believers in your church - they will all not love one another as John commands in his first letter, but they will rather love themselves, trying to prove that they are worthy of respect and acceptance.

You will see this in the choices people make regarding their jobs, courses of study and how they choose to spend their money. The examples are numerous!

In your counselling, you will have to identify the meaning people ascribe to life and try to understand their actions and words against that background.

You will also have to teach them about the true meaning of life and help them to redirect their lives according to this true meaning.

Life in the Presence of God

In the previous lecture, we ended by discussing the Biblical idea of the meaning of life. It was pointed out that a good grasp of the true meaning of life will help you to counsel others effectively.

In this lecture, we continue with the second important issue regarding the task of the pastor in counselling the individual believer, pointed out in the Introduction to Lecture 1: the believer's journey through life.

The Believer's Journey through Life

Justification and Regained Meaning

It is in the context of man forever seeking to restore his own paradise that the saving work of Jesus Christ receives its full meaning. In Christ, those who believe are restored to the right relationship with God: that of being his servant and his representative.

COUNSELLING AND JUSTIFICATION:

The key word in all Christian counselling is justification. Without the justification of sinners in Jesus Christ, there is no sense in doing any counselling.

Why? Because in Christ, on the basis of the blood he has shed for us, every believing sinner is restored to being accepted and worthy - in the sight of God. This means that the believer does not do good, work hard, earn money or gain power in order to be accepted and respected (by God or other people), but, precisely because he is already accepted and respected by God, he does good and works hard.

This is a complete reversal of man's motivation in life - it is, in fact, a reversal of what happened at the fall.

Because of being justified in Christ, life itself regains its original meaning:

- To glorify God instead of oneself;

- To serve God and other people in selfless love;

- To work as God's loving and caring representative in this world, thereby reflecting his glory;

- To worship him and have fellowship with him, thereby giving him his due.

Once this fact has been accepted by whoever comes to you to seek your help in counselling, the way is open for you to proceed with your work, because the basic foundation is right.

You may freely reprove, challenge, encourage and teach within the context of a shared belief regarding the meaning of human life. You will not be tempted to seek for solutions promising happiness or other good feelings, power, wealth, liberation or anything else.

Your guide and goal in all counselling are to bring the believer to practical decisions (repentance, changed behaviour) on the basis of his restored relationship with God, the restored meaning of his life in Jesus Christ.

Your goal is to help believers to change their lives (in all their relationships, in everything they do, say and think) in accordance with their most basic identity - that of being "the image of God".

When confronted by people, their problems and their attempts at solving these problems, let this be the test you apply:

- Are their lives and their attempted solutions in accordance with their being "in the image of God", or do they serve only to strengthen their selfish quest for acceptance and respect?

- What can you do to change their thinking and their actions, so that they will then live renewed lives as servants of God and their fellow men, people who truly glorify God in everything they do?

- Sanctification and Growing Meaning

In the last paragraph, we spoke of a regained sense of the meaning of life on the basis of justification in Christ. This is not enough, however, for providing you with a clear knowledge of what counselling is all about. If you stick with justification, you have only the foundation of the house, and not yet the walls themselves. More has to be said.

After justification comes sanctification.

- Sanctification is nothing else than being continually transformed into the image of Christ, who is himself, as Son of God, the image of God.

- Sanctification is to become more and more like Christ in righteousness, holiness and knowledge of God's will.

- To be sanctified is to be changed into a person reflecting the face of Christ himself so that whoever looks at you, will recognize Christ in you.

Again it has to be said that counselling does not have as its ultimate goal the happiness, self-expression, liberation, development or dignity of man, but only conformity to the image of God, by means of becoming more and more like Christ!

Christians have to walk the path from justification to their eventual glorification in the new heaven on the new earth. They know that they will reach their final destination because they know themselves to be secure in God's love and faithfulness.

The route they follow is that of obedience to Christ their Lord, through the power given to them by the Holy Spirit.

Along the way, there will be many obstacles preventing true obedience, not the least of which is a lack of moral courage. However, the true believer will always get back on his feet again, in the power of the Spirit, with his eyes fixed on Jesus Christ.

The final result will be a continuous growth towards spiritual maturity by being constantly renewed in thoughts, feelings, desires and actions.

Paul speaks of spiritual maturity in Christ in Ephesians 4:13-16.[28]

Through their individual and joint service, the church (both as individual members and as a unity) experiences growth. Like any growth, the growth of the church culminates in maturity, but in the case of the church, it is a special kind of maturity: it is the maturity of the perfectly balanced character of Christ![29]

Moreover, it is a maturity that brings stability in the face of many false teachers and heretics (2 Timothy 3:16), not only those who proclaim false doctrine, but also those who preach a wrong way of life!

As a pastor, you will be expected to "speak the truth in love", in order to guide those who are misguided, to teach those who are ignorant, and to help those who are weak. Only then will you be helping along the faithful on the long road of growing up in Christ, until the day when they will be made perfect.

The sharing of personal brokenness forms the backbone of the Christian counselling process because people in real need, experiencing real hurt will find it difficult to identify with superheroes. They would rather prefer to share themselves with those who are authentic enough to admit that "they had been there before". One of the reasons why Paul became a real leader was because of the fact that he had a clear grasp on his personal brokenness.[30] (Rom 7:18-25)

The counsellor must also not be perceived as the person with the answers. Paul was equally clear on this when he stated that we are looking in a mirror in this life and that we will never understand everything but that it will be revealed to us one day[31]. (1Cor 13:12) No human being no matter how well qualified and spiritually intact will ever qualify as the bearer of answers or solutions to the pain, needs and questions of others. Christ is the only answer because Christ is the only healer. The true and honest counsellor is only becoming involved in a spiritual quest to find Christ's answer to the need and hurt and pain suffered by the brother or sister coming for help.

Presented with this route-map of the Christian life, you will know what to do and say to believers who come to you for help.

You will teach and reprove, encourage and help, always keep in mind the journey from justification, through sanctification, to glorification.

Life in the Presence of God.

All of the above will of course only make sense and be truly helpful if both pastor and believer share a deep sense of living life in the immediate presence of God, or what some Bible translations call "in the sight of God."

Any meaningful sense of the true purpose of life will only have effect in the context of life consciously lived in the presence of God. In the same way, the absolute need for continuing sanctification, and the deep longing for eventual glorification will only arise from being conscious of living life in the presence of God.

The imperative inherent in any call for a change in one's ways is also only meaningful against the background of a God who cannot be deceived and who knows everything - even the deepest and most secret desires of our hearts.

You may well ask how it is that we live our lives in such close proximity to God. As in everything else, the answer is Jesus Christ. He is Immanuel - God with us!

- In Christ, who lives in us through his Holy Spirit, God has come to make his dwelling in our hearts. It is for this reason that the apostle Paul can speak of the church and every believer individually as the temple of God (Ephesians 2:22; 1 Corinthians 3:16).

Also, we are present before the throne of God in the person of Jesus Christ, who is the pledge of our future life with God (1 Corinthians

15:20). In truth, we already dwell at the right hand of God in fellowship with Christ!

It will be helpful to review your study of Psalm 139 at this point. Take special note of the awesome responsibility of living life so openly before God!

The true believer will find in this Psalm a source both of deep comfort and joy, on the one hand, and extreme distress, on the other hand:

- Comfort because of the knowledge of being enclosed on all sides by the loving presence of God;

- Distress because he knows that every sinful thought or desire is completely open before God, even if nobody else knows about it.

The Psalm speaks in glowing terms of a God who is at work in this world, whose purposes are being achieved in human lives, who is concerned with and cares about people. One of the most important consequences of this is the profound knowledge that, whatever our circumstances or our problems, God is involved! This knowledge is the source of the greatest comfort both for you as a counsellor and for those you counsel.

It makes all the difference in the world between merely listening with compassion, and being able to offer real hope. It also makes all the difference between a merely humanistic or man-centred approach to counselling and an approach that honours God and puts him first.

Such an approach, which honours God, is also consistent with the words of Jesus in the Sermon on the Mount when he told his disciples first to seek the kingdom of God and his righteousness, and not their own comfort or solutions to all their own problems. Rather, he emphasised that a life free of superficial cares and unsolved problems will be the share of those who place God first (Matthew 6:33-34).

The mechanisms of human behaviour

Once you know why you actually engage in counselling as part of your pastoral ministry, your next objective is to find out how you do it. In order to do so, we will first discuss the nature and mechanisms of human behaviour.

It is a foundational aspect of the Bible's revelation that man was created without sin, and that sin entered into the world and into human lives through the arrogant disobedience of Adam and Eve. It is an equally foundational fact that everything mankind has ever done after the fall has been tainted, even motivated, by sin and sinful objectives and desires. There has never been a perfect human being again, with the exception of Jesus Christ.

In your counselling, you will meet with all kinds of sinful behaviour - some quite consciously sinful, others unconsciously so. You will also meet with people suffering from the effects of other people's sinful behaviour, or from the results of living in a broken world. Whatever the face of what you meet, the common denominator will always be the same: sin, sin and once more sin!

The question is how to deal with this sin:

- Do you simply point it out, and demand change with authority that comes naturally to a servant of a Lord who is primarily Judge?

- Or do you simply show all the compassion you can muster, as a good disciple of a Lord who knows nothing of righteousness and justice?

- Or is there perhaps another alternative?

The first alternative mentioned above is based on the view that sin is a sin, and there is neither a reason nor an excuse for committing it. Your only task is to find it, repent of it and change your behaviour.

The second alternative assumes that man is merely the innocent victim of evil forces greater than himself. Because he cannot fight them, your task is to comfort him in the suffering caused by the terrible injustice of being dragged into a monumental battle with which he is not at all concerned.

There is, however, a third alternative, which includes both the emphasis on God's righteous demand for moral obedience and Christ-like compassion for people who suffer terribly at the hands of their own sin and that of other people.

This alternative presupposes a clear understanding of the mechanisms of human behaviour, the effects of sin on this behaviour and the way out of this difficult situation.

Your position as a counsellor is not one to be envied: you have to represent God's viewpoint of demanding moral purity, as well as his all-encompassing love for his sadly, misled creatures.

You dare not enter into any counselling without that deep compassion for sinful, suffering people which we find embodied in the person and work of Jesus Christ - a compassion which is not, however, a mere love for people, but love which has as its only goal the glory of God and the eternal well-being of those you counsel.

It is sometimes a lot easier to help people with problems to meet their immediate needs than to present them with God's goals for life - as long as their anxiety and pain are eased.

It is sometimes also easier merely to be extremely righteous about everything, and go about finding sin and demanding change, without any real concern for the living, complex person sitting in front of you - as long as God's honour is maintained.

Neither, however, represent a true example of the task of the Christian pastor's counselling objectives, namely to bring people to an understanding of the consequences of salvation in Christ and of a life lived to the glory of God. The previous lectures in this module should have made that abundantly clear.

Let us now devote ourselves to trying to understand the intricate mechanism of human behaviour.

The Need for Significance and Security

The most basic need of any human being is to be recognized as being worth something - it is a need for what we call personal worth:

- When other people recognize your personal worth, they treat you with respect, listen to what you have to say, recognize your efforts to do something worthwhile with your life, and generally treat you as a sane, normal human being, equal to themselves in all respects.

- When they do not, however, recognize your personal worth, you will be treated as a less-than-human being, with no respect and no attention for what you are saying or doing. You will be passed by in all their plans as if you are not important enough to be remembered, mentioned or included in their plans. The only time you will be noticed is when you represent an obstacle to the fulfilment of their plans.

We now have to make a further distinction. The need for personal worth can be divided into two further distinct needs, both of which together when fulfilled, constitute a sense of personal worth.

These two further needs are:

- The need for significance:

This need is a very complex one, and consists of:

- the need for purpose and meaning in your life,

- the need for being (or doing something) important,

- the need for being adequately skilled or gifted for what you have to do,

- and the need for making a difference in the world through what you do.

- The need for security: this need consists of:

- the need for unconditional acceptance by other people (especially group-acceptance),

- the need for a close, loving relationship with those nearest to you (wife/family)

- the need for consistent expression of this acceptance and love.

Before the fall, Adam and Eve also had the need for personal worth, as expressed in the need for significance and security. They were created with these needs - it was part of what made them human.

These needs were automatically provided for by God, who gave them:

- all the purpose and meaning they ever wanted,

- important work to do,

- the skills they needed to do it,

- and the possibility of making a difference in their world (guiding creation towards fulfilment by, for instance, naming the animals and working the garden of Eden!)

- They also had the unconditional love and acceptance of God and each other

- and this love and acceptance were constantly expressed in their mutually close and trusting relationship.

After the fall, however, everything changed. By cutting themselves off from God, thereby also cutting themselves off from the task He has given them to do and from each other, they lost the fulfilment of their most basic needs:

- they no longer had a sense of purpose or meaning;

- their work became difficult and meaningless - their only aim now was to survive;

- they no longer had the skills or the interest to do their new work properly;

- their work no longer included the possibility of making any difference in the world - it became menial, unimportant and boring.

- They lost God's love and acceptance and now feared instead of trusted Him;

- they became strangers to each other, hiding their nakedness in shame, blaming each other for their changed circumstances.

Yet their needs for significance and security did not disappear - only the original means for fulfilling them were no longer available!

- They now turned to each other, expecting their husbands or wives to provide them with the love and everlasting security of unconditional acceptance which only God could give.

They were bound to be disappointed!

- When their husbands and wives disappointed them, they turned to other men and women and committed adultery again and again, in order to find the love and acceptance they so desperately needed.

They were bound to be disappointed!

- They turned to money and power to make them feel important and waged war after war to increase their wealth and power.

They were bound to be disappointed!

- They started to tell lies and boast about their skills and abilities because they had to gain respect at all costs.

They were bound to be disappointed!

- They turned to violence and fraud in their need to change the world which no longer satisfied them.

They were bound to be disappointed!

- The comfortable relationship with nature which had existed before the fall now became a terrible struggle for survival and mastery over the forces of nature. Man became plagued by droughts, famines and floods. He was threatened by fire, wind and water.

Because man no longer believed in God, he turned to spirits, forefathers and animist forces for the help he needed to survive in a hostile world.

He was bound to be disappointed!

Wherever man turned, he invented substitute fulfilments for his needs. They were substitutes because they were not the means intended by God. They were found, invented or imagined by man himself - and none of them could satisfy as God had once satisfied!

These needs are very powerful forces, shaping and determining people's behaviour. You will not understand a man's adultery unless you understand his need for unconditional acceptance and respect from a woman. You will not understand a young man's materialism unless you understand his deep need for feeling important and being respected by others.

You will not understand a student's perfectionism unless you understand that he has learnt that good marks can earn love, respect and acceptance from others. You will also not be able to free these people from their driving needs unless you understand and are able to show them how their deepest needs can and should be fulfilled by Christ Jesus.

True Significance in Jesus Christ

Our true significance depends upon who we are in Jesus Christ, who makes everything new - including our most basic identity as human beings. We will eventually come to feel significant as we have an eternal impact on people around us by ministering to them (all Christians, not only pastors, should minister to all people!).

Whatever our circumstances (whether poor or rich, young or old, weak or strong), because we belong to Christ through the saving work he has done, we can enjoy the thrilling significance of belonging to the Ruler of the universe who always has a job for us to do. This gives importance, purpose and meaning to our lives, and grants the opportunity for making a difference in the world around us.

Christ also equips us for the work he calls us to do, by giving us the gifts of the Spirit (Ephesians 4:7-16). We can, therefore, know that we are always adequately skilled for whatever we have to do in His service.

As we mature by becoming more and more like Christ, we will more and more experience the true significance which is ours through belonging to and serving the Lord Jesus Christ.

True Security in Jesus Christ

As is the case with our significance, our true security also depends on our new identity in Jesus Christ. God has seen us at our worst and, unlike any human beings we know who would reject us immediately when they see us like that,

He loved us to the point of giving the life of his Son in a hideous suffering. This is the kind of love we can never lose! We are completely acceptable to God, regardless of our behaviour, because our acceptability to God depends only on Jesus' acceptability to God and on the fact that Jesus' death was regarded as full payment for our sins.

Because of this new position in Christ, nothing can happen to me that my loving Father does not allow, and I will experience nothing he will not enable me to handle.

When problems do come and I feel alone, insecure and afraid, I will fill my mind with the security-building truth that at this moment an all-powerful, loving, personal, infinite God is absolutely in control, and that I am safe in the intimate relationship I have with him through Jesus Christ. In this knowledge, I find absolute security!

However, no matter how true these things are, no matter how much security we derive from the fact that we are acceptable to God through Jesus Christ no matter what we do - we are not entitled to a careless living. We remain responsible to God for how we live! Sin remains sin, and it is not fitting that we who are new in Jesus Christ should live like the old, sinful people we once were (Ephesians 4:17-32).

Our lives have to be holy, not because we can earn God's love in that way, but precisely because we already have God's love in Jesus Christ!

Without God-in-Christ, people will always develop alternative strategies for feeling significant and secure[32] , However, these always fail at a certain point, because they were never intended for that purpose - they deliver neither lasting significance, nor lasting security! Instead, they often become big dangers to our sense of significance and security!

Our money, our children, our families turn against us and become sources of terrible worry. Our marriages and careers fail, our houses are robbed or burned, our political parties desert us, and our plans do not realize. Instead of comforting us, they destroy us, as all idols eventually do.

Only in Jesus Christ do we find true and lasting significance and security.

The Role of the Conscious Mind

Now that you understand the basic motivating forces behind most of human behaviour, we will continue with the actual mechanisms of the specific things we do every day of our lives. The most important elements we will consider are:

- the roles of the conscious and unconscious minds,

- the basic direction of our hearts,

- the role of the will and

- the role of emotions.

As conscious human beings, we constantly think about things happening around us. Not only do we think about them, but we also evaluate them: we ascribe a positive or negative value to them, saying that they are either good or bad.

It is this evaluation we make of things happening around and to us, which influences our feelings or emotions - not the things themselves! Mere events cannot influence our emotions. Our subjective evaluation of events can and do influence our feelings, and these feelings, in turn, influence our behaviour.

Incidentally, it is this same conscious mind which Paul refers to in Romans 12:2, when he says that our minds have to be renewed - the way in which we think about and evaluate our world - if we are to become more and more like Christ!

An example could illustrate this nicely. When you go to bed one evening, your next day is all planned. Your corn is ready to be harvested, and you plan to get up very early the next morning, even before sunrise, to go and bring in the harvest. However, when you wake up before dawn the next morning, it is raining very hard, and there is no way that you could either go out and work in the rain or bring in wet corn. As soon as you store it, it will rot! You are also afraid that the whole harvest will rot in the fields if the rain continues too long.

The result of that will be poverty and hunger - too bad even to think of! Your family will think that you are not able to provide for them, and they will reject you. Other people will also lose respect for you when they see your hungry children begging for food. So you become terribly depressed because you are worried sick about these things.

Notice how your evaluation of the rain is negative, and that it is this evaluation which makes you feel depressed, because your need for security (the idea that you must always provide sufficient food, or else your family and other people will reject you) and your need for significance (your ability to feed your family) is being threatened!

You could also have argued as follows: yes, it is raining, and yes, I cannot harvest the corn. It is true that it might rot if the rain doesn't stop soon, and that poverty and hunger might be the result of it. My family might think less of me, and other people might scorn me because of my inability to feed my children.

However, it is also true that God is my Father, and that he provides me and my family with everything I need. My significance and security rest in Christ, not in my family's evaluation of me. Therefore, this rain is not the best thing that has ever happened to me, but it is also not the worst disaster ever to come over me. Therefore, I can be concerned, but also have great peace! I need not feel depressed!

Notice that in this line of reasoning, you have changed your evaluation of the circumstances (the rain), based on a different set of ideas regarding your sense of security and significance. As a result, you do not experience the same feelings you would otherwise have experienced!

Now the question is: why did you evaluate the rain as negative in the first place? This will become clear as we consider the role of the unconscious mind.

The Role of the unconscious Mind:

———

The source of those basic assumptions which people firmly and emotionally hold about how to meet their needs for significance and security is often located in the unconscious mind. This means that we are mostly not consciously aware of the things we regard as being able to provide for our needs for significance and security.

Unconsciously, we all look to something or someone other than God to give us the good things in life. These can be our parents, our forefathers, our government, our money, luck, forces of nature, and so on. All of these are used by Satan when he teaches us that our needs would be met if only we had money, food, luck, love, pleased forefathers, satisfied gods, fertile wives or any of the other things we depend on.

These basic, unconscious beliefs determine our evaluation of events, things and people. If events or people fit our unconscious beliefs, we evaluate them positively, if not, negatively. In terms of our example above, we could say that the basic, unconscious belief was that we must always be able to provide sufficiently for our families, or else they will reject us.

As a result, the rain threatens our need for security and significance and is, therefore, bad. (At other times, when the rain was necessary for our crops to grow, we would have given it a positive evaluation!) It is evident that not God, but our own ability to provide for our families, are trusted to make us feel good, to give us a sense of significance!

Another example: a young wife loves her husband very much, and he loves her. However, after five years of marriage, she has not become pregnant. She knows that her husband expects of her to provide him with lots of children, but there is nothing that she can do about it. She is afraid that her infertility will cause her husband to reject her, and she becomes terribly depressed. She now fears her husband and withdraws from him.

Her basic assumption, which she unconsciously holds, is that she must provide her husband with lots of children in order for him to love her (the need for security), and in order for other people to respect her as a good wife (the need for significance). She now evaluates her childlessness, her physical appearance, her identity as a woman and her relationship with her husband as negative, because of this basic, unconscious belief, and she becomes depressed and withdrawn.

Her trust was in her ability to have children because that would have made her secure and significant. However, once she has learned that not her ability to have children, but rather Jesus Christ is the source of her security and significance, she can once again become a good and loving wife - even without children!

If we are to help solve people's painful problems, we will need to help them become conscious of and absolutely honest about these deep, unconscious motivating factors. This is not so easy because all people are masters of self-deception. You will also find many people who will be able to give you all the right answers about where they should find their security and significance. They answer you, however, with their conscious minds, while their lives are being determined from their unconscious minds. Their behaviour will often show that they indeed do not find their significance and security in Jesus Christ.

It is for this reason that both you as a counsellor and the person you counsel need the help of the Holy Spirit, who alone can investigate the deepest secrets of our minds and hearts, and convince us of the deception we force on ourselves (compare Jeremiah 17:9-10).

The Basic direction of the Heart:

In Scripture, the heart is indicated as the deepest core of a person, the source of all sin and/or holiness (Proverbs 4:23).

- It is in the heart that the deep conviction that "I serve myself, not God or anybody else" is rooted.

- It is also the heart that is changed when God renews us in Jesus Christ, with the new basic conviction that "Henceforward I will serve God alone, not myself or anybody else."

Because of this basic orientation towards or away from God, the heart determines the basic direction of our lives: whether we will be faithful to God or live lives of sin.

If we choose to live for ourselves and not for God, which we all naturally do in our sinful nature, our deepest needs will never be met. In deciding against God and for ourselves, we cut off the only source of true security and significance. We will search for substitutes all our lives, but they will never completely satisfy - no substitute is ever as good as the real thing.

On the other hand, if we are brought to decide for God and against ourselves by serving Christ and becoming more and more like him, we are linked to the source of true security and significance.

This kind of attitude is summarized by the following expressions in the New Testament:

- "not as I will, but as you will" (Matthew 26:39);

- "I have been crucified with Christ, and I no longer live, but Christ lives in me" (Galatians 2:20);

- "whoever loses his life for me will find it" (Matthew 16:25).

This new life of close union with Christ, in which Christ himself takes over complete control over our hearts and lives and in which our own will is dissolved in the will of Christ, will result in the following course of events:

- our hearts will have a new direction,

- with the result that our unconscious minds will eventually be cleaned or renewed by the Spirit;

- this will, in turn, result in a different evaluation of circumstances, events and people in our conscious minds

- and helped by the conscious application of the truth of Scripture.

As long as our unconscious minds have not been completely renewed (and they will never be absolutely free of sinful impulses until the day we die), obedience to Scripture through the power of the will, will often have to override our instinctive reactions to circumstances, events and people, for the sake of being obedient to Christ. This will help us to evaluate these things not against the background of our sinful unconscious minds, but rather against the background of the truth of Scripture.

Continued obedience to Scripture - which is the same as obedience to Christ - will also in the long run aid the transformation of our unconscious minds!

The Role of the Will:

———

Not all behaviour is simply the result of unconscious factors and influences. People can also choose how to behave, as when we decide that we will not loose our temper even though we are provoked.

However, the decisions we make regarding our behaviour are normally only made from a limited range of possibilities. These possibilities for behaviour are only those that we actually understand to be sensible. For example, when I tell you to jump into a raging river in flood and swim across it, you will think I have lost my mind. However, if I add that an angry lion is chasing you, you will immediately see the sense of jumping into the river and swimming as fast as you can!

As long as you do not understand the good sense of a possible course of action, you will ordinarily not choose to follow it. Once you do understand that there is a good reason to do something, however, you will accept it as a possibility you could willingly choose to follow.

Now, you could spend all your time and energy trying to persuade people to change their sinful behaviour. However, they will not willingly choose to obey as long as they do not understand the sense of what you are proposing.

Remember that their sinful behaviour serves a purpose: it provides them with pleasure or a sense of personal worth!

There is a reason for what they do. You will only make obedience to Christ a viable option to them once they understand that true joy, true security and significance and true peace are to be found in Jesus Christ alone!

Only when people really understand the person and work of Christ as the basis for true life, will they be willing to choose a life in obedience to him.

Of course, not all the responsibility for this will be in your hands. Christ himself will also bring people to understanding through Scripture and the work of the Holy Spirit. You are a tool in the hands of Christ: it is your task to explain Scripture to people who need a new direction in their lives.

Always remember that obedience to Christ does not automatically follow correct understanding. It is an old (and wrong!) Western idea that knowledge guarantees virtue.

Our understanding merely determines the range of options we can choose from. The will now choose responsible behaviour consistent with the teachings of the Bible because this choice is recognized as being the most meaningful one from the range of possibilities.

This is not always easy - it often involves teeth-gritting effort to choose to behave as we should, because this choice goes against the grain of everything we have ever consciously or unconsciously believed to provide us with a sense of personal worth, comfort, joy or pleasure (compare Paul's struggle as reported in Romans 7!).

Apart from a clear exercise of the will, there will be no consistent obedience! It is really a matter of exercise - the more you do it, the easier it will become.

The Role of Emotions:

Some people believe that if you walk with the Lord and confess all your sins, you will never have bad feelings. Others believe that we will always experience bad feelings simply because we are human and live in a broken world, but we should never allow other people to know that we experience them - especially not if we are Christians!

It is clear from the Bible that not all bad feelings are morally wrong. Some feelings can hurt badly, but they still exist in us together with feelings of deep peace and joy. Christ himself cried at the grave of Lazarus (John 11:33, 38) - and nobody can claim that his sorrow was sinful!

You might have experienced this with the death of a loved one: you are terribly sad and the thought that the dead person will never return hurts badly, while your longing and loneliness seem to tear you apart. However, if you know that the person was a true believer, you will also know that he or she is now with Christ, in heavenly joy, and this knowledge will give you peace and joy! The bad feelings exist together with the good ones.

There are, however, also bad feelings originating in sinful living and thinking. The two examples mentioned above, of the threatened harvest and the childless woman, prove this point. These feelings have to be identified, their sources checked, and they should then be dealt with.

How do we distinguish between "good" bad feelings and "bad" bad feelings?

As a general rule of thumb, we could say that:

- Any feeling which is mutually exclusive with compassion, blocks the development of compassion or prevents the expression of compassion, involves sin.

- Compassion is the foundational feeling of a life centred in Christ.

- It is the feeling or emotion belonging to the life-attitude of love, which the apostle John discusses in his first letter.

- A good barometer of our fellowship with Jesus Christ is the level of compassion we feel for a lost world and a suffering church.

You have now seen how people will devise strategies for satisfying their needs for significance and security. These needs and the ways people have identified to have them satisfied most often operate at an unconscious level. They do, however, influence the way we think about and evaluate the world around us, with all its events, people and circumstances.

This thinking or evaluation takes place in the conscious mind through conscious thinking. In its turn, our conscious evaluation of the world around us determines the way we feel about it - whether good or bad.

The strategies we devise to satisfy our need for personal worth develop along the lines of the basic direction of our lives, as determined by the direction of our hearts - whether toward or away from God.

People whose hearts are directed to God will depend on God for the fulfilment of their need for personal worth, and this basic dependence will influence the way they evaluate the world and the events of their lives. In their conscious evaluation of the world, the Bible plays a guiding role.

People whose lives are not centrally directed towards God through their hearts, but rather at themselves, will devise surrogate strategies to have their needs satisfied. They will depend on their own abilities, wealth, power and so forth to build security and obtain significance in their lives. Anything which threatens them in this process will cause them to react negatively, causing bad feelings and sinful behaviour.

It is also very important to understand that the person who is competent to counsel others must never perceive his or her experience as a solution or a guideline to the needs of others. The fact that the counsellor had been in a place of discontent before or that God has helped him or her in a specific way only serves as a witness or beacon of hope but it never becomes the template or perfect example on how God's unique solution to the needs of the person seeking help will finally become a reality. God's answer to the personal needs of others must never be limited to the counsellor's personal experiences and insights. Counselling is much more a joint quest towards discovering God's unique and specific solution to the need of the person seeking guidance. This is true because of troubles and adversities, no matter how negative, has a unique application in each believer's life and always work for the good when used by God to build character into a person. It is, therefore, important to always keep in mind that suffering and emotional distress form part of God's character building process and that this process is experienced in a unique manner by each person. [33] (Rom 5:3-5)

DEPRESSION IN GENERAL

First recorded description of depression:

- Hippocrates in the 4th century provided the first description of depression
- He called it "melancholia"
- Believed it was caused by excess black bile in the brain

Types of Depression

Reactive depression.

Endogenous depression.

Primary and secondary depression.

Reactive Depression (as a reaction to something)

This comes as a reaction to some real or imagined loss or trauma like the death of a loved one.

Endogenous Depression (as a result of imbalance in the body chemistry)

It is also called autonomous and sometimes psychotic depression and is more likely to arise spontaneously from within.

Primary and Secondary Depression

Primary depression occurs by itself while secondary depression comes as the side effect of some medication, the influence of one's diet, or the result of an illness like cancer, diabetes, or even influenza.

Depression is a common but complicated condition, difficult to define, hard to describe with accuracy, and not easy to treat.

The Bible and Depression

Depression is a clinical term that is not discussed in the Bible even though the condition appears to have been common. Psalm 69, 88 and 102, for example, are songs of despair but notice that these are set in the context of hope. In Psalm 43 David expressed both depression and rejoicing. Job, Moses, Jonah, Peter and the whole nation of Israel experienced depression (Job 3; Num 11:10-15; Jonah 4:1-3; Ex 6:9; Matt 26:75). Elijah wanted to die (1 Kings 19).

These examples, accompanied by numerous references to the pain of grieving, show the realism that characterises the Bible. It is a realistic despair contrasted with a certain hope. The biblical emphasis is less on human despair and more on belief in God and the assurance of abundant life in heaven, if not on earth (Ps 34:15-17; 103:13,14; Matt 5:12; 11:28-30; John 14:1; 15:10; Rom 8:28).

The Causes of Depression

The Christian counsellor needs to take note that it is not true for example, that:

- Depression always results from sin or a lack of faith in God
- All depression is caused by self-pity
- It is wrong for a Christian to ever be depressed
- Depressed feelings can be removed by spiritual acts

Christians like everyone else get depressed and the causes can be grouped into two major categories:

- The genetic-biological causes or physical reasons.
- The psychological-cognitive causes or emotional reasons.

The genetic-biological causes

Depression often has a physical basis:

- Lack of sleep
- Insufficient exercise
- Side effects of drugs
- Physical illness
- Women experience depression as part of a monthly pre-menstrual syndrome (PMS)
- Some are victimised by postpartum depression following childbirth

The psychological-cognitive causes

Background and family causes

Some evidence suggests that childhood experiences can lead to depression in later life:

- Children who had been separated from their parents
- Teenagers in conflict with their parents
- People from unstable homes
- College students with negative opinions about their families
- Stress and significant losses

Stress makes us feel threatened when we experience a loss:

- Loss of an opportunity, a job, health, possessions etc.
- Divorce, death or prolonged separations
- Learned helplessness

Depression can occur when we encounter situations over which we have little or no control:

We learn that our actions are futile no matter how hard we try nothing can be done to relieve our suffering reach a goal, or bring change

Cognitive causes (or "thinking" causes)

How a person thinks often determines how he or she feels:

If we think negatively, we see only the dark side of life

Depressed people can show negative thinking in three areas:

- They view the world and life experiences negatively
- They view themselves negative, inadequate, unworthy which in turn leads to self-blame and self-pity
- View the future in a negative way - looking ahead they see continuing hardship, frustration, and hopelessness

Anger

An old and widely accepted viewpoint suggests that depression comes when anger is held within and turned against oneself

Many children are raised in homes where the expression of anger is not tolerated.

Some attend churches where all anger is condemned as sin

Other people are convinced that they shouldn't even feel angry, so they deny hostile feelings when these do arise

Sin and guilt

S in and guilt can lead to depression

When a person feels that he or she has failed or done something wrong, guilt arises and along with it comes self-condemnation, frustration, hopelessness, and other depressive symptoms

The Effects of Depression

- Unhappiness and inefficiency.
- Physical illness.
- Low self-esteem and withdrawal or separation from others. Depression and feelings of loneliness walk hand in hand.
- Suicide.

Unhappiness and inefficiency

Depressed people frequently feel "blue", hopeless, self-critical, and miserable. The result:

- They lack enthusiasm
- They are indecisive
- They sometimes have little energy

Life thus is characterised by:

- Inefficiency
- Underachievement
- Increased dependence on others

Physical illness

Depression including the sadness that comes with grief or loneliness tends to suppress the body's immune system. Depressed people, therefore, are more likely than others to get sick.

Low self-esteem

When a person is discouraged, unmotivated there often is low self-esteem, self-pity, a lack of self-confidence, and the strong desire to get away from other people. Social contacts may be too demanding and the depressed person may not feel like communicating.

Suicide

Suicide and suicide attempts are often seen among teenagers, people who live alone, the unmarried (especially the divorced), and persons who are depressed. For some suicide attempts are:

- An unconscious cry for help
- An opportunity for revenge (get them back)
- A manipulative gesture designed to influence some person who is emotionally close

Counselling and Depression

Because of the depressed state of mind, the counsellor must reach out verbally, taking a more active role:

- Make optimistic reassuring statements
- Share the facts about how depression affects people
- Patiently encourage individuals to talk
- Ask questions
- Give periodic compliments
- Gently share the Scripture (without preaching)
- Try to avoid confrontation

As the counsellor talks about the depression, you should:

- Listen attentively
- Watch for evidence of anger, hurt, negative thinking, poor self-esteem and guilt
- Encourage individuals to talk about those life situations that are bothersome
- Watch for talk about losses, failures, rejection

In counselling the depressed, some the following approaches can be helpful:

Dealing with the causes

Counselling will be easier if you can find the psychological and spiritual causes that produce the symptoms. Try to discover through questioning and careful listening what might be producing the depression.

Dealing with thinking

To change feelings we must change thinking. The counsellor tries to help the individual evaluate their:

- Expectations
- Attitudes
- Values
- Assumptions

Help individual sees which of these are:

- Unrealistic
- Non-biblical
- Harmful

Since these kinds of thoughts often are well entrenched, sometimes coming from a lifetime of thinking, it may take repeated efforts to help people re-evaluate and change their attitudes toward life and themselves.

Dealing with inactivity

Depressed people often lack the energy or the motivation to take actions that will deal with the problem. For many, it is easier to stay in bed or to sit alone brooding and thinking about the miseries of life.

Gently, but firmly, you may need to push the depressed person to:

Take action

- Get involved in daily routines, family activities, and recreation
- When the individual does take action try to give encouragement and compliments.
- Dealing with the potential for self-harm
- Suicide is one action that is contemplated by many depressed people.

Be alert for example to the following:

———

- Talk of suicide
- Feelings of hopelessness
- Indications of guilt feelings and worthlessness
- An inability to cope with stress
- Excessive concern about physical illness
- A sudden and unexplainable shift to a happy, cheerful mood (which often means that the decision to attempt suicide has been made)
- Knowledge regarding the most effective methods of suicide
- A history of prior suicide attempts (those who have tried before, often try suicide again)

Counsellors should not hesitate to ask whether or not the individual has been thinking of suicide. Such questioning gets the issue out into the open and lets the individual consider it rationally. If a person is really determined to commit suicide the counsellor may delay this action, but in time the individual will try again.

Preventing Depression

- Trust in God who gives strength and is able to supply – Phil.4:11-13
- Expect discouragement, our faith will be tested – James 1:2-3
- Be alert to depressed-prone situations – holidays, Christmas, etc.
- Learn to handle anger and guilt
- Challenge thinking – positive self-talk
- Finding support – try not to be alone
- Reaching out – helping others
- Encourage physical fitness

Anxiety

Definition

Anxiety is an inner feeling of uneasiness, concern, and worry that is accompanied by heightened physical reactions like sweating excessively, hyperventilating (quick breathing) etc.

Types of Anxiety

- Normal anxiety.
- Neurotic anxiety.
- Moderate anxiety.
- Intense anxiety.
- State anxiety.
- Trait anxiety.
- Post-traumatic stress disorders.
- Anxiety disease.

Normal anxiety

- Most often, this anxiety is in line to the danger - the greater the threat the greater the anxiety
- It is anxiety that can be recognised, managed, and reduced, especially when circumstances change

Neurotic anxiety

Neurotic anxiety involves intensely exaggerated feelings of helplessness and dread even when the danger is mild or non-existent

Many counsellors believe this anxiety cannot be dealt with rationally because it may arise from inner conflicts that are not conscious

Moderate anxiety

Moderate anxiety is one of those types that can be desirable and healthy. Often it motivates people to avoid dangerous situations.

Intense anxiety

This is more stressful and hinders performance skills

State anxiety

- It often comes quickly and has a short duration
- It is an acute, relatively brief apprehensive reaction that comes to all of us from time to time

Trait anxiety

Trait anxiety, in contrast, is a persistent, ever-present, ingrained emotional tension

It is seen in people who appear to worry all the time

Often it causes physical illness

Post-traumatic stress disorders

This is an extension of intense stress such as rape, violence, and involvement in a serious accident, kidnapping, or natural disasters such as floods or earthquakes.

Anxiety disease

This is a term used to describe sudden, terrifying, severe panic attacks. Increasing evidence now indicates that the root is biological.

The Bible and Anxiety

In the Bible anxiety is used in two ways:

Anxiety as health concern

Anxiety as a realistic concern is neither condemned nor forbidden Although Paul could write he was not anxious about the possibility of being beaten, cold, hungry, or in danger, he said that he was anxious about the welfare of the churches (2 Cor. 11:28 and Phil. 2:20)

Anxiety as fret and worry

Anxiety as fret and worry may have been in the psalmist's mind when he wrote that "anxiety was great within me," and that God's consolation brought joy (Ps. 94:19). Jesus taught that we should not be anxious about the future; we have a Father who will provide (Matt 6:25-34)

Anxiety as fret and worry comes when we turn from God and assume that we alone are responsible for handling problems

There is nothing wrong with honestly facing and trying to deal with the identifiable problems of life

To ignore danger is foolish and wrong. But it is also wrong and unhealthy to be immobilised by excessive worry

Causes of Anxiety

- Threat.
- Conflict.
- Fear.
- Unmet needs.
- Individual differences.

Threat

Sometimes anxiety arises because one's life is threatened. More often we feel threatened (and therefore anxious) because of:

- Danger – crime, war, unexpected illness, etc
- Loss of self-esteem – think we are not competent, feel threatened
- Separation from others – death, divorce, etc
- Undermining of our values – fail to get a promotion, etc

Conflict

Two tendencies for conflict are:

- Approach and Avoidance

There are three basic kinds of conflicts:

Approach-Approach Conflict

You may be faced with two dinner invitations on the same night and become anxious because you cannot decide what to do

Approach-Avoidance Conflict

A desire to do something and not to do it - An offer for a new job, to accept bring more money, but you have to move, etc

Avoidance-Avoidance

Two alternatives, but both may be unpleasant – a painful illness versus an operation that can be painful

Fear

<hr>

Many different factors play a role in causing us fear: failure, the future, war, rejection, sexual intimacy, success, taking responsibility, conflict, sickness, death, loneliness, change and a host of other real or imagined possibilities.

Unmet needs

There are six suggested fundamental needs that should be met in order to prevent anxiety

- Survival - the need to have continual existence, knowing where one is going
- Security - the need for emotional and economic stability
- Sex - the need for intimacy
- Significance - the need to do something and be worthwhile
- Self-fulfilment - the need to achieve fulfilling goals
- Selfhood - the need for a sense of identity or being someone

Individual differences

People react differently to anxiety-producing situations. Some people are almost never anxious while other seems anxious all the time.

The Effects of Anxiety

- Physical reactions.
- Psychological reactions.
- Defensive reactions.
- Spiritual reactions.

Physical reactions

It is common knowledge that anxiety can produce ulcers, headaches, skin rashes, backaches, and a variety of other physical problems.

Psychological reactions

Anxiety can reduce productivity (so we don't get much done), hinder interpersonal relations, dull the personality, and interfere with the ability to think or remember.

Defensive reactions

When anxiety builds, most people unconsciously rely on behaviour and thinking that dull the pain of anxiety and makes coping easier. These defensive reactions are seen often in counselling. They include ignoring the feelings of anxiety; pretend the anxiety-producing situation does not exist, convincing oneself that there is "nothing to worry about."

Spiritual reactions

Anxiety can motivate us to seek Gods help that might be ignored otherwise

At the same time anxiety can drive people away from God at a time when He is most needed

Counselling and Anxiety

Anxious people often make others anxious, including the counsellor who is trying to help.

To counsel anxious people, therefore, the counsellor must first be alert to his or her own feelings.

- Recognising the counsellor's own anxieties.
- Calming tension.
- Showing love.
- Identifying causes.
- Making interventions.
- Encouraging action.
- Giving support.
- Encouraging a Christian response.

Recognising the counsellor's own anxieties

Ask the question "What in this situation is making me anxious?"

Calming tension

Counselling is unlikely to be effective if the counselled is too tense to concentrate. To deal with this tension, let the counselled see that you are a calm, caring, and reassuring person.

Showing love

Love is self-giving and moves toward others, but fear shrinks away from them. The Bible states that perfect love drives out fear (1 John 4:18).

Identifying causes

The sensitive counsellor does not tell the counselled to "stop being anxious." Most of us get no help from the well-meaning, but naïve Christian, who proclaims that worry is a sin that can be stopped at will.

Making interventions

Anxiety differs from person to person yet in spite of these differences; anxiety can be dealt with in various ways:

- Biological intervention - anxiety is treated medically
- Behavioural intervention - behaviours are taught - to be more relaxed
- Environmental intervention - change one's lifestyle, relationship, career

Encouraging action

The purpose of counselling is not to eliminate all anxiety. Instead, the goal is to assist counselled individuals in discovering the sources of their anxiety. Then they must learn to cope.

Giving support

A supportive relationship is imperative in counselling anxiety.

Encouraging a Christian response

A better approach is to focus on activities and thoughts that indirectly reduce anxiety. The Bible shows how this can be done and in so doing it gives a formula to be shared with counselled individuals:

- Rejoice - Phil. 4:4
- Be gentle - Phil. 4:5
- Pray - Phil. 4:6
- Think - Phil. 4:8
- Act - Phil. 4:9

Preventing Anxiety

Trust in God

Learn to cope – admit fears, talk with someone, seek help

Keep things in perspective – keep a realistic perspective

Reach out to others

Conclusion

Anxiety warns people of danger and motivates us to take action. When it creates panic or immobilizes individuals the anxiety is dangerous.

Jesus put all of this in perspective when he spoke about worry in the Sermon on the Mount. God knows about our needs and anxieties. Jesus said if we give Him first priority in our lives, we can rest assured that our needs will be supplied and that there will be no need to be anxious. This is a message that makes Christian counselling unique.

ALTERNATIVE MODEL

Pastoral Psychology

147

The treatment of Depression and Anxiety Disorders

Before anyone can begin with treatment or with understanding the need of the person suffering, one need to first determine what depression is and what the signs and symptoms are.

What is depression?

Encarta gives the following definition of the word DEPRESSION:

Depression (psychology), is a mental illness in which a person experiences deep, unshakable sadness and diminished interest in nearly all activities.

People also use the term depression to describe the temporary sadness, loneliness, or blues that everyone feels from time to time.

In contrast to normal sadness, severe depression, also called major depression, can dramatically impair a person's ability to function in social situations and at work.

People with major depression often have feelings of despair, hopelessness, and worthlessness, as well as thoughts of committing suicide.

Some psychologists are promoting that depression is an immense feeling of sadness. This feeling can last for a short period of time, but can also last for very long periods of time.

When depression is not treated it can last for years and cause immense damage to the person suffering from it.

A person suffering from depression need to know that depression is an illness like diabetes and others and that it needs to be treated before the positive change will take place.

Signs of depression:

1. A feeling of sadness. Normal sadness can touch anyone and is normally of a short period of time. The sadness coupled with depression is a longer lasting one.

2. A feeling of worthlessness.

Symptoms of depression:

The most common symptoms are:

1. A depressed and irritable outlook most of the time and mostly every day.

2. Extremely reduced interest in pleasurable daily activities.

3. Changes in appetite, leading to an increase or decrease of weight.

4. Sleep disturbances leading to little or excessive sleeping.

5. Agitation or slowing down.

6. Loss of energy or fatigue.

7. Feelings of worthlessness or guilt.

8. Decreased ability to concentrate and to make decisions.

Other symptoms:

9. Excessive introspection.

10. Anxiety.

11. Crying for no apparent reason.

12. Nightmares.

13. Cold sweat.

14. Becoming a perfectionist.

15. Thinking about death and even about suicide.

Variation between different groups:

Having any of these symptoms does not mean that one suffers from depression. It is only after most of these symptoms are prevalent that such a deduction can be made.

Male versus Female depression sufferers:

Depressed women are more likely to experience feelings of guilt, weight gain, anxiety and eating disorders are sleeping disorders than men.

Older adults also suffer a more frequent feeling of emptiness than younger sufferers would.

Some well-known people who were suffering from depression:

Winston Churchill - British Prime Minister.

Billy Graham - Evangelist.

Peter Sellers - Actor.

Vincent van Gogh - Artist.

Sigmund Freud - Psychologist.

Mark Twain - Author.

As can be seen from the above-mentioned list, depression can attack anyone. No-one is immune to it.

According to Research, about 19 million American suffer from depression.

Reasons for suffering from depression:

1. Bereavement because of the loss of a loved one.

2. Postpartum depression during or just after a woman has given birth.

3. Seasonal Disorders normally developing during winter.

4. Bipolar Depression, previously known as manic depression disorder associated with mood swings.

5. Medical conditions like Parkinson's disease and HIV.

6. Certain medication used muscle relaxants, steroids and medication for diabetes.

7. Reaction to toxins and metals like lead, pesticides and petrol.

8. Intoxication withdrawal from substances like alcohol and other drugs.

Types of depression:

There are 2 types of depression presenting in sufferers, either:[34]

Endogenous depression

This depression is summed up as coming from within the sufferer. It is important to note that this type of depression does not have to do with external influences, yet the depression will inevitably lead to a negative response to interaction with others.

This type of depression is normally genetically inherited.

The person will have a greater tendency towards suicide. In one recorded case a sufferer of 3½ years tried to commit suicide.[35]

The main cause o this type of depression is the over-production of the chemical substances noradrenalin and serotonin. These chemicals control the synaptic contact between the nerve cells in the brain. Should there be interference in the synapses the cells will transmit fewer messages to other cells.

Exogenous depression. (Formally also known as Reactive depression.)

This can again be subdivided between:

a. Uni-polar depression

Sufferers of this type of depression present with a singular focus of negative feelings.

This type of depression is characterized by the following symptoms:

- Found in 2 – 3 times more in women than in men.
- The person has a negative outlook on life.
- He will have sleep disturbances.
- He will be more prone to suicide than someone that suffers from bipolar depression.
- He will present with a low energy drive.
- He will withdraw from personal contact with others around him.

b. Bipolar depression

Sufferers of this type of depression present with two extreme poles of feelings, being positive and joyous the one moment and changing to negative and depressed the next moment.

This type of depression was also known as manic depression.

In most cases, this type of depression can be medically treated by means of lithium salts.[36]

This type of depression is characterized by the following symptoms:

- An equal distribution between males and female sufferers.
- The person will be clamorous and monomania.
- He will apparently not need any sleep as he continuously feels energized.
- The person's chances of suicide during the manic stage are very low.

Treatment of the depression sufferer:

- The most general method of treatment is called cognitive therapy. It is a short-term treatment that can have a long-term effect.
- Therapeutic sessions of three months have a much greater success rate than talk therapy that has taken place over a period of years.[37]
- The relapse rate is also much lower than other types of therapy, while the longtime effect of treatment is far better than any other therapy, again emphasizing the importance of this type of therapy.
- The use of this type of therapy also protects the sufferer from the indications and contra-indications presenting in medication.[38]

Statistics that need to be considered:

Research has demonstrated that roughly half of individuals receiving competent psychotherapy show measurable improvement by the end of the eighth weekly session.

This increases to 74 percent after the twenty-sixth weekly session.

Of all the people treated for depression, up to 80% have presented with improvement either through medication or counselling.[39]

(In some cases a combination of the two procedures are needed to attain success. This is especially beneficial when the sufferer does not respond to any individual therapy and is found in about 15% of those suffering from depression.)[40]

The most successful method of counselling consists of short-term therapy, normally lasting between 12 to 16 sessions.[41] It should also not be discounted that God can heal any person of any illness at any time.

Having been given a background as to the causes and symptoms of depression the following will have to be remembered by the person treating the sufferer:

- In order for you to counsel effectively, you will need to know how problems develop, or else your counselling sessions will be no more than warm, friendly and compassionate conversations, full of good intentions. Alternatively, you will just say: "That is sinful! You must repent and change! Here are the Scriptures to read to help you."

- Neither of these approaches really constitute effective counselling, because neither take into account the full complexity of human behaviour, especially of sinful behaviour. Let us therefore first have a look at how problems develop.

Needs and Wants

———

We have already discussed every person's need for personal worth, or the need for security and significance. We will now call this need our primary personal need, which should be distinguished from primary physical needs of food, clothing and shelter.

The fulfilment of these primary personal needs is absolutely essential for the personal well-being of any human being. In most cases, people attempt to meet these needs through things like money, fame, recognition, promotion at work, a new home, a good marriage, better looks, an improved slimmer figure, business success, nice kids and good friends, even an effective ministry.

We will now call these things, through which people try to meet their primary personal needs, secondary personal needs or wants. These wants eventually become independent of the needs they were originally intended to satisfy, and assume the role of primary needs:

- Money is then no longer intended for survival but becomes a need in itself.
- Sex is no longer a means for achieving intimacy but turns into what would seem to be a primary need for pleasure or power, crying out to be fulfilled.
- Approval, originally intended to provide a deep sense of security, becomes a ruling passion in one's life.

You as a counsellor will have to learn to recognize the hidden primary personal need behind the secondary needs stressed by people and show them how their personal needs can truly be met.

These needs or wants are called secondary or acquired because we do not absolutely need them to be whole persons who live biblically. We may want them passionately to the point where their absence provokes a non-sinful, legitimate and excruciating pain, but they are not essential for being a whole person! I can live a deeply meaningful and personally whole life without satisfying these wants, even if my life may be filled with anguish because of their absence.

All I need for rational, responsible, obedient and committed living, for a whole and meaningful life, is for my primary personal needs to be met in Jesus Christ. The apostle Paul is a very good example of such a person: He had neither freedom nor good health; he was a short little man, with a bad personal history; many people disliked him (but as many loved him like their own brother); he spent long years in prison and often had to run away from angry crowds of people. Yet he remained committed to serving Christ, always singing joyful songs of praise to God and testifying to a deeply meaningful life (Acts 16:25; Philippians 1).

His need for security and significance was fully met in Jesus Christ!

Many of these secondary needs or wants present us with a sinful pattern of living: a constant striving for recognition and approval makes a life of simple service almost impossible; a promiscuous life, where sex is always looked for in new places, with new people and in new ways, is of course never a holy life of moral purity; a life spent in collecting more and more wealth eventually turns into ordinary greed.

Most of these needs reflect a self-centered life, with a heart which is not directed at God but at my own selfish wants. You need no proof to convince you that such a life is not life as God intended it!

Our primary needs of security and significance can never be taken away from us - we were created with them.

However, our secondary or acquired needs can be changed, even cancelled out:

- if they create a problem

- and if there is a problem-free route to meet the same primary needs the acquired needs were designed to meet.

Motivation

Motivation is the drive or urges to meet my needs - it is that which forces me to fulfil my needs of security and significance, even if it requires a large amount of personal energy.

The direction in which I apply this motivating force (also called goal-oriented behaviour) is completely determined by what I think will meet my primary personal needs (also called a basic assumption). This conviction is called a strategy for meeting our needs. The world (our parents, friends and cultural environment), our own flesh (our sinful nature) and the devil all work together to teach us false strategies for meeting our personal needs.[42]

People generally experience emotional problems when their strategies for reaching their goals fail, or when their goal-oriented behaviour turns out to be ineffective. There are three basic reasons why people fail to reach their goals:

- the goals are unreachable, in which case people often feel guilty or inadequate when they fail to reach their goals;

- external circumstances get in the way, in which case they feel resentment and unreasonable anger;

- they are afraid of failure, and then try too hard, in which case they experience anxiety.

They will then often come to you asking you to help solve their frustration or to cure their depression, or to help them get rid of an overwhelming sense of emptiness and meaninglessness.

It should by now already be clear to you that these strategies for meeting our primary personal needs for significance and security are sinful because we put something else in the place of Jesus Christ.

It would, therefore, also be wrong for you to help people achieve more successful goal-oriented behaviour as long as their strategies are still sinful. Your task is not to relieve their frustration or depression or sense of emptiness, while at the same time making them more effective sinners, but rather to teach them correct strategies for reaching legitimate goals so that they can learn to serve God as obedient servants!

First and foremost the sufferer should be pointed to the Word of God.

Each session **MUST** be started and concluded by praying for the Lord's guidance.

The Apostle Paul was faced with numerous trials and tribulations, yet he exclaimed not once, but twice: "Rejoice in the Lord!"[43] Two verses later he also exclaimed: "Be anxious for nothing."[44]

The person should be pointed out that by not keeping his eyes upon the Lord he is directly opposing the Biblical command of not being anxious but by trusting in the Lord.

The person is directed to the principle that we should love our fellow man because God loves us, an important part in the way we interpret Theology. God loves us with all of our mistakes, therefore, we should also love our fellow man as well.[45]

It is important to speak truth from the Word of God. God's Word gives comfort.

Unbelieving counsellors usually define their task as the responsibility for individual people's welfare - to make them feel good. Christian counsellors, however, are also concerned with people's welfare, but they redefine "welfare!"

We want to introduce changes which will draw a person closer to God, whether the immediate feelings caused by this are good or bad. Remember, the Christian counsellor is in the unique position of advising people to live in a way which may increase the burden of life and even make it seem unbearable!

But what do you actually try to change?

You could start by trying to change people's primary personal needs, but you will remember that we have said that these needs are part of the most basic human identity. We were all created with these needs by God, and they cannot be taken away.

You could also argue that it is the motivation that has to be changed - what we have called the driving force behind all action intended to meet our primary personal needs. However, it is not the force itself that causes problems, but rather the way in which the force is applied and the direction in which it is applied. Motivation as such cannot be taken away because without it people would never act!

The next possibility is to change the basic assumptions regarding how our primary personal needs can be met. If our basic assumptions conform to the revealed truth of Scripture (namely that our primary personal needs can and should only be met in Jesus Christ), all the problems mentioned above can be avoided. No emptiness, no despair, no frustration, resentment or anxiety will be experienced; we will also not need all the emergency remedies we usually employ to ease the pain and frustration for lives not lived according to God's plan.[46]

Transformation, then, depends on renewing not our feelings, nor our behaviour, nor our circumstances, BUT OUR MINDS! Remember Romans 12:1-2!

As a Counsellor one will listen to the person and not judge or criticize and will treat the person without pessimism and anger.

Should anger manifest it need to be dealt with immediately.

It is very important to listen to and to look for suicidal tendencies. The person can sometimes say that he does not see a future for himself anymore and wants to end his life. The Councillor would then have to act decisively and encourage the person to speak about his fears and reasons for his feelings.

In most cases where anger is involved, the person will be angry because of either other people, or with himself.

An atmosphere of openness needs to be established where the issue is mentioned by name, not referring to "it".

The person should also be encouraged by speaking in a normal voice when referring to the issues that need to be dealt with.

He should not speak about his issues in a hushed voice. By doing this the issue is again coming to the fore and can be dealt with.

The Councillor should resist the temptation to give advice or to complete sentences. The person must be afforded the opportunity to be heard and to be able to formulate his feelings. A grieving person longs to be heard.

It is also important to be patient with the person.

Lead the person to express his emotions.

Be honest towards the person.

Although there are times when strong and direct confrontation is necessary in counselling, there are other times when gentle support, encouragement, listening, reflection, clarification and acceptance of feelings are what is needed.

Counselling is not like a recipe, in which you follow a certain number of steps in the correct order, and then achieve automatic success.

It is much rather a relationship of mutual trust and deep, compassionate caring. Even so, a certain number of indications or directions can be given, in order to effectively structure this relationship.

Identify Problem Feelings

Most people in need of counselling will present themselves with a feeling, difficult circumstances or problem behaviour. Your first objective is to identify problem emotions. This gives you a starting point, from which you could proceed with the counselling session.

Most important, try to decide whether these problems feelings are one of the following:

- guilt,
- resentment,
- anxiety,
- despair or
- a feeling of emptiness (cf 2.2 above).

When the person you are counselling begins with difficult circumstances, you should also ask how he or she feels about these circumstances. The feelings you identify are helpful guides towards a diagnosis for the specific problem related to goal-oriented behaviour.

In the same way, if the person comes to you with problem behaviour, try to identify the feelings associated with this behaviour. Go through all the areas of the individual's life: work, family (marriage, children, parents, brothers and sisters), sexual activity, religion and church-related activity, education and money. In all of these, look for problem feelings.

Identify Goal-Oriented or Problem Behaviour

As soon as you have identified problem feelings, you can then proceed to trace goal-oriented behaviour on the basis of these feelings. You will remember that we have indicated how specific ways in which goals are not reached lead to different kinds of problem feelings.

By working backwards from these feelings, you should be able to trace the problem with the goal(s) set by the person.

For instance, if a woman experiences deep resentment towards her husband, you will expect that the problem will be one of the external circumstances preventing her from reaching her goal.[47]

He would perhaps always be making jokes about her physical appearance, while she desperately needs him to approve of her physical appearance, in order to feel accepted and secure.

She is forever working hard at maintaining her good figure, dresses carefully and spends a lot of time on her physical appearance. Her husband's jokes, however, prevent her from reaching this objective, and she, therefore, experiences resentment towards him.

In your counselling, you will now deal not with her resentment, but rather with her goal-oriented behaviour, namely of working towards earning her husband's acceptance of herself by means of his approval of her physical appearance.

Identify Problem Thinking (= Basic Assumptions)

Once you have identified this goal-oriented behaviour, you should next ask yourself what kind of basic assumption is presupposed in this kind of behaviour.

In the example mentioned above, it would seem as if the woman needs her husband's approval of her physical appearance in order to feel accepted and, therefore, secure in her relationship with him. This is her basic assumption: her security in life depends on her husband's acceptance of her physical appearance.

Change the Problem Thinking (= Basic Assumptions)

This step is perhaps the most difficult of all. You will now need to convince your counselled that his or her thinking/basic assumption is indeed wrong.

You will then have to teach him or her the correct, biblical way of meeting our personal primary needs of security and significance. This is the most difficult part because the basic assumption with which a person operates is often so deeply rooted, that simply explaining an alternative will not change it.

You will first have to investigate where this basic assumption was learned. In the case of our example, the woman could simply have been indoctrinated by society's insistence on physical beauty as a prerequisite for a loving relationship.

She could also have learned it from her mother, who had the same basic assumption. Perhaps she used to be overweight as a little girl, and she was mocked because of it. Whatever the case may be, it would help to find out where this basic assumption came from.

Because the basic assumption is often a very emotional subject, primarily because it was learnt in emotionally charged circumstances, expression and acceptance of these emotions will often help the counselee to relax with you and consider what you have to say.

You will also have to understand that people will be threatened if you suddenly pull down their defences. The woman in our example has learned that she can earn acceptance and avoid ridicule if she works hard at her physical appearance. She is safe as long as she presents a good image.

However, if you suggest that this is the wrong way for her to protect herself from ridicule and rejection, she will have to let go of it and allow herself the risk of being exposed to rejection and emotional pain. She will, of course, resist this! You will have to be very encouraging and supportive during this phase of counselling.

Back to our primary goal: to change the problem thinking.

The counselee will now have to be taught the correct assumption, in accordance with the teachings of Scripture.

This will often involve the rather mechanical process of repeating it over and over in the mind whenever the old bad feelings return until it becomes natural to think only of the correct assumption.

Secure a Commitment

Merely learning and repeating the correct assumption is good but not enough. The counselee will also have to commit herself to acting in a way consistent with this new basic assumption.

This will often involve acting against one's feelings, simply because one knows that this is indeed the obedient thing to do!

Plan and Carry out Biblical Behaviour

Once the counselee is committed to acting in a way consistent with the newly learned, biblical basic assumption, her future behaviour will have to planned in some detail. A new discipline of behaviour will have to be set up because consistent behaviour over a long period of time will also change the counselee's way of thinking or the basic assumption.

It is one thing to agree with a basic assumption, but quite another for that assumption to be fixed so deeply in one's mind that one's acts on it almost without thinking!

Identify Spirit-Controlled Feelings

Once the new discipline of a life in radical obedience to Christ has been achieved over a period of time, the counselee should also start to experience feelings of deep peace and quietness, with a sense that life is once again "whole." These feelings should be pointed out to the counselled so that they can be consciously enjoyed!

The person needs to be assured of acceptance, which is lacking in his current feeling of self-judgment and sometimes even hatred.

This acceptance can be summed up as "facing the truth."

Often the person will be confronted with shame and guilt. He needs to be assured that the Councilor has accepted him as he is.

It is important to let the person understand that the Councillor is "there" for him and that he wants to understand his feelings.

Being "there" for the person does not mean that he must be pitied. It is important to assist him but feeling pity for him can lead to an increase in depression.

The first step in the healing process would be to find the source of the depression. This could have been brought on by self-guilt, recurring patterns of interpersonal relationships, unresolved grief, etcetera.

A recommended way of finding and dealing with the problem would be for the counsellor to draw a circle, divide it into parts and to write the losses in this.

When the elements are seen, it transforms the depression into something concrete that can be seen and managed.

Normally the source can be identified through this exercise. Should the source not be manifested, it would mean that a deeper source exists that need to be explored even further.[48]

The person can also be encouraged to write down his feelings. This will again lead to him expressing himself, handling the issue and to bring anger to the front.[49]

It could be necessary to lead the person to the point of expanding his assertiveness and not to be the peacemaker normally taking all the blame just to keep peace in the family.

The person should also be made aware of negative stimuli that could trigger a bout of depression.

This is also applicable where the person is requested to give possible answers to the problems that are facing him. He should be encouraged to seek positive answers to his questions.

The person needs to be lead not to be excessively negative in this approach. Normally people suffering from depression will catastrophize when trying to problem-solve. When he presents with a negative feeling he is lead to examine those thoughts, finding out how accurate they are and to consider alternative outcomes.

He should also be lead to adapt new ways of handling his feelings and his depression.

The person will also be encouraged to change his habits in the following areas:

- Establishing normal full night sleeping habits
- Eliminate or reduce the intake of alcohol and caffeine
- Exercising
- Improving his diet

- He should be encouraged to again follow a "regular" schedule of routine.
- Discourage the sufferer from being alone for long periods of time as loneliness leads to him thinking about his depression again and can lead to an onslaught of negative thoughts.
- Help the person to set "bite size" or short term goals. After each completed the goal the person will have a positive experience which in turn will lead to lessening the negative thoughts located within the person.

The family also needs to understand why he is changing the areas mentioned above.

The person needs to be encouraged to visit his doctor as well as tests can be done to address concerns he has, or to determine if the depression is not being brought on by some sort of deficiency.

Finding that the source of depression is family based then the counsellor will need to refer the husband and wife to attend marriage or family counselling.

Open communication must be encouraged amongst the family members.

It is, therefore, important to encourage the person to have an honest relationship with his children. (Should there be children.)

The person will at some time during the counselling be faced with grief, sorrow or guilt. This will have to be handled very carefully by the Councillor.

The person will be shown how to distinguish between false guilt true guilt.

The person needs to be brought to the process of regaining perspective.[50]

He should again be brought to again gain perspective of his life.

He needs to be shown that life has meaning and will have meaning again.

He will be shown that he had joy in his life and that he will again have joy after dealing with his depression.

He will be shown that the losses that one face and the gains one enjoyed will all come together as ingredients that will make up his experience in life.

The person will be helped to accept the grace of God as well as His forgiveness for the transgressions that have led to the feeling of depression.

He will be told that God's grace is sufficient for us [51] and that He will forgive all our sins if we ask His forgiveness.[52]

Bibliography:

Adams, J.E. 1979. A Theology of Christian Counselling: More Than Redemption. Grand Rapids: Zondervan

Adams, J.E. 1980. Marriage, Divorce and Remarriage in the Bible. Grand Rapids: Zondervan

Adams, J.E. 1986. The Biblical View of Self-esteem, Self-love, Self-image. Eugene: Harvest House.

Brammer, Lawrence M (Ed). 1977. Therapeutic Psychology. Prentice-Hall Incorporated

Brennan, PA et al. (2000). Developmental Psychology, 36, 759-766

British Journal of Psychiatry June 1987, Vol. 150 by J.L. Cox, J.M. Holden, R. Sagovsky

Chapin, Shelly. 1992. Counsellors, Comforters & Friends. Victor Books

Crabb, L.J. 1985. Effective Biblical Counselling: How to Become a Capable Counsellor. London: Marshall Pickering

Lam, dr. Raymond W. 2000. Depression Information and Resource Centre distribution pamphlet

Lexapro. 2002. Depression Information for you. Medical pamphlet for the product – LEXAPRO, Forest Laboratories

Luoma, I et al. (2001) Journal of the American Academy of Child & Adolescent Psychiatry, 40,1367-1374

Prinsloo, Jean 1998. Hoop vir depressielyers. Johannesburg: Baruk

Shields, Brooke. 2005. Down came the rain: My journey through postpartum depression Hachette Books

Vericker Tracy et al. (2010) "Infants of Depressed Mothers Living in Poverty: Opportunities to Identify and Serve" Brief of The Urban Institute

http://www.beatricedegelder.com/publications.html

https://books.google.co.za/books?id=Ab9u_AyU9aUC&pg=PA363&lpg=PA363&dq=Kiserud+et+[1]

https://books.google.co.za/books?id=vPbSAwAAQBAJ&pg=PA174&lpg=PA174&dq=Niebyl+et+a U4L1iCQ&hl=en&sa=X&ved=0ahUKEwjy9q6wiO_SAhXjBsAKHQq-

---

1. https://books.google.co.za/
books?id=Ab9u_AyU9aUC&pg=PA363&lpg=PA363&dq=Kiserud+et+al.,+2004&source=b
l&ots=J6CbBzlKPm&sig=3KwvljID750LsnKJyOU5DPBcPFs&hl=en&sa=X&ved=0ahUKE
wi37tjshu_SAhUHBMAKHR7ABiwQ6AEIIjAD#v_43ec3e5dee6e706af7766fffea512721_on
epage_6cff047854f19ac2aa52aac51bf3af4a_q_43ec3e5dee6e706af7766fffea512721_Kiserud_0
bcef9c45bd8a48eda1b26eb0c61c869_20et_0bcef9c45bd8a48eda1b26eb0c61c869_20al._0bcef
9c45bd8a48eda1b26eb0c61c869_2C_0bcef9c45bd8a48eda1b26eb0c61c869_202004_6cff047
854f19ac2aa52aac51bf3af4a_f_43ec3e5dee6e706af7766fffea512721_false

AI4Q6AEIIjAC#v=onepage&q=Niebyl%20et%20al.%2C%202010&f=false

[2]

https://books.google.co.za/
books?id=zigp-66vq0MC&pg=PA330&lpg=PA330&dq=Saletu+et+al.,+20

[3]

---

2. https://books.google.co.za/

books?id=vPbSAwAAQBAJ&pg=PA174&lpg=PA174&dq=Niebyl+et+al.,+2010&source=bl

&ots=OPbYbKfQbx&sig=m6tvwDS89Qi4fuW0VW1-

U4L1iCQ&hl=en&sa=X&ved=0ahUKEwjy9q6wiO_SAhXjBsAKHQq-

AI4Q6AEIIjAC#v_43ec3e5dee6e706af7766fffea512721_onepage_6cff047854f19ac2aa52aac5

1bf3af4a_q_43ec3e5dee6e706af7766fffea512721_Niebyl_0bcef9c45bd8a48eda1b26eb0c61c8

69_20et_0bcef9c45bd8a48eda1b26eb0c61c869_20al._0bcef9c45bd8a48eda1b26eb0c61c869_

2C_0bcef9c45bd8a48eda1b26eb0c61c869_202010_6cff047854f19ac2aa52aac51bf3af4a_f_43

ec3e5dee6e706af7766fffea512721_false

3. https://books.google.co.za/

books?id=zigp-66vq0MC&pg=PA330&lpg=PA330&dq=Saletu+et+al.,+2001+postpartum+

depression&source=bl&ots=M9sh24rXv3&sig=_HCaPBXzGyjxnkvRmOL85gA1xDk&hl=e

n&sa=X&ved=0ahUKEwifm4vGiu_SAhUlIsAKHfYMCuQQ6AEIHTAA#v_43ec3e5dee6e

706af7766fffea512721_onepage_6cff047854f19ac2aa52aac51bf3af4a_q_43ec3e5dee6e706af7

766fffea512721_Saletu_0bcef9c45bd8a48eda1b26eb0c61c869_20et_0bcef9c45bd8a48eda1b2

6eb0c61c869_20al._0bcef9c45bd8a48eda1b26eb0c61c869_2C_0bcef9c45bd8a48eda1b26eb0

c61c869_202001_0bcef9c45bd8a48eda1b26eb0c61c869_20postpartum_0bcef9c45bd8a48eda

1b26eb0c61c869_20depression_6cff047854f19ac2aa52aac51bf3af4a_f_43ec3e5dee6e706af77

66fffea512721_false

https://books.google.co.za/
books?id=Vd54AgAAQBAJ&pg=PT381&lpg=PT381&dq=Tronick+and[4]

http://www.bing.com/videos/watch/video/brooke-shields-discusses-her-struggle-with-postpartum-depression/6d4s5kv

http://courses.washington.edu/evpsych/
Morrison-et-al-prefs&menstrual-cycle-ASB2009.pdf

http://ecommons.luc.edu/cgi/
viewcontent.cgi?article=1513&context=luc_diss

https://en.wikipedia.org/wiki/Postpartum_depression

http://www.health.com/health/condition-video/
0,,20193997,00.html

http://jme.endocrinology-journals.org/content/38/3/383.full

http://www.mededppd.org/pdss.asp

http://www.ncbi.nlm.nih.gov/pubmed/20483973

https://www.ncbi.nlm.nih.gov/pmc/articles/PMC2612082/

https://www.ncbi.nlm.nih.gov/pmc/articles/PMC2819576/

---

4. https://books.google.co.za/
books?id=Vd54AgAAQBAJ&pg=PT381&lpg=PT381&dq=Tronick+and+Field,+1986&source=bl&ots=F0RqIovvHO&sig=fE5njaZSurEs8XpZDD-RLxW_bZI&hl=en&sa=X&ved=0ahUKEwiSiIi3je_SAhVnBsAKHbrJCucQ6AEIKjAC#v_43ec3e5dee6e706af7766fffea512721_onepage_6cff047854f19ac2aa52aac51bf3af4a_q_43ec3e5dee6e706af7766fffea512721_Tronick_0bcef9c45bd8a48eda1b26eb0c61c869_20and_0bcef9c45bd8a48eda1b26eb0c61c869_20Field_0bcef9c45bd8a48eda1b26eb0c61c869_2C_0bcef9c45bd8a48eda1b26eb0c61c869_201986_6cff047854f19ac2aa52aac51bf3af4a_f_43ec3e5dee6e706af7766fffea512721_false

https://www.ncbi.nlm.nih.gov/pmc/articles/PMC2684038/

https://www.ncbi.nlm.nih.gov/pubmed/9489170

http://patient.info/doctor/patient-health-questionnaire-phq

http://www.pitt.edu/~jeffcohn/biblio/CohnTronick1989.pdf

http://scholar.google.co.za/
scholar_url?url=https://www.researchgate.net/profile/
Peter_Cooper12/publication/
10780199_Controlled_trial_of_the_short-_and_long-
term_effect_of_psychological_treatment_of_post-
partum_depression_I_Impact_on_maternal_mood/links/
569b679008ae748dfb0e39d8.pdf&hl=en&sa=X&scisig=AAGBfm1bOmhqc
N0ac6RTfOq3A&nossl=1&oi=scholarr&ved=0ahUKEwjAo9imhu_SAhXr(

http://www.youtube.com/watch?v=BloACoqVs1o&feature=related

http://www.youtube.com/watch?v=FjJuN9Qfr0I

http://www.youtube.com/watch?v=u5DprqJSk20

[1] http://jme.endocrinology-journals.org/content/38/3/383.full

[2] http://www.beatricedegelder.com/publications.html

[3] https://www.ncbi.nlm.nih.gov/pmc/articles/PMC2612082/

[4] http://scholar.google.co.za/scholar_url?url=https://www.researchgate.net/profile/Peter_Cooper12/publication/10780199_Controlled_trial_of_the_short-_and_long-term_effect_of_psychological_treatment_of_post-partum_depression_I_Impact_on_maternal_mood/links/569b679008ae748dfb0e39d8.pdf&hl=en&sa=X&scisig=AAGBfm1bOmhqoNQnBqIN0ac6RTfOq3A&nossl=1&oi=scholarr&ved=0ahUKEwjAo9imhu_SAhXrCsAKHV

[5] https://books.google.co.za/books?id=Ab9u_AyU9aUC&pg=PA363&lpg=PA363&dq=Kiserud+et+al.,+2004&s

[6] https://en.wikipedia.org/wiki/Postpartum_depression

[7] http://courses.washington.edu/evpsych/Morrison-et-al-prefs&menstrual-cycle-ASB2009.pdf

[8] https://books.google.co.za/books?id=vPbSAwAAQBAJ&pg=PA174&lpg=PA174&dq=Niebyl+et+al.,+2010&soU4L1iCQ&hl=en&sa=X&ved=0ahUKEwjy9q6wiO_SAhXjBsAKHQq-AI4Q6AEIIjAC#v=onepage&q=Niebyl%20et%20al.%2C%202010&f=false

[9] http://ecommons.luc.edu/cgi/viewcontent.cgi?article=1513&context=luc_diss

[10] https://www.ncbi.nlm.nih.gov/pmc/articles/PMC2819576/

[11] https://books.google.co.za/books?id=zigp-66vq0MC&pg=PA330&lpg=PA330&dq=Saletu+et+al.,+2001+postp

[12] http://www.ncbi.nlm.nih.gov/pubmed/20483973

[13] http://www.health.com/health/condition-video/0,,20193997,00.html

[14] https://www.ncbi.nlm.nih.gov/pmc/articles/PMC2684038/

[15] The law, P.L. 2006, c. 12 amends N.J.S.A. 26: 2-175 et seq. and took effect on October 10, 2006.

[16] Adapted from DSM IV-TR, Washington, D.C.: American Psychiatric Association; 2000.

[17] Vericker Tracy et al. (2010) "Infants of Depressed Mothers Living in Poverty: Opportunities to Identify and Serve" Brief of The Urban Institute

[18] https://www.ncbi.nlm.nih.gov/pubmed/9489170

[19] http://www.who.int/mental_health/prevention/suicide/lit_review_postpartum_depression.pdf

[20] http://scholar.google.co.za/scholar_url?url=https://www.researchgate.net/profile/Peter_Cooper12/publication/10780199_Controlled_trial_of_the_short-_and_long-term_effect_of_psychological_treatment_of_post-partum_depression_I_Impact_on_maternal_mood/links/569b679008ae748dfb0e39d8.pdf&hl=en&sa=X&scisig=AAGBfm1bOmhqoNQnBqToT-N0ac6RTfOq3A&nossl=1&oi=scholarr&ved=0ahUKEwjAo9imhu_SAhXrCsAKHVGXC

[21] Brennan, PA et al. (2000). Developmental Psychology, 36, 759-766

Luoma, I et al. (2001) Journal of the American Academy of Child & Adolescent Psychiatry, 40,1367-1374

[22] http://www.pitt.edu/~jeffcohn/biblio/CohnTronick1989.pdf

[23] https://books.google.co.za/books?id=Vd54AgAAQBAJ&pg=PT381&lpg=PT381&dq=Tronick+and+Field,+1986&sc

[24] http://www.mededppd.org/pdss.asp

[25] http://patient.info/doctor/patient-health-questionnaire-phq-9

[26] Taken from the British Journal of Psychiatry June, 1987, Vol. 150 by J.L. Cox, J.M. Holden, R. Sagovsky

[27] The thought of harming myself has occurred to me.

Yes, quite often

Sometimes

Hardly ever

Never

[28] In this passage it is interesting to note how Paul links the work of the pastor (among others) to the process of building the congregation by equipping the members for.

[29] In the context of the counselling session, we will define maturity as:

- Immediate obedience to Christ as Lord in any specific situation;
- Long-range character growth in conformity to Christ as image of God.

[30] *Rom 7: 18-25*

I know that nothing good lives in me, that is, in my sinful nature. For I have the desire to do what is good, but I cannot carry it out. For what I do is not the good I want to do; no, the evil I do not want to do – this I keep on doing. Now if I do what I do not want to do, it is no longer I who do it, but it is sin living in me that does it. So I find this law at work: When I want to do good, evil is right there with me. For in my inner being I delight in God's law, but I see another law at work in the members of my body, waging war against the law of my mind and making me a prisoner of the law of sin at work within my members. What a wretched man I am! Who will rescue me from this body of death? Thanks be to God - through Jesus Christ our Lord! So then, I myself in my mind am a slave to the law of sin.

[31] *1Co 13:12*

For now we see in a mirror, dimly; but then face to face: now I know in part; but then shall I know fully even as also I was fully known.

---

[32] (= WORTHY).

[33] *Rom 5:3-5*

Not only so, but we also rejoice in our sufferings, because we know that suffering produces perseverance; perseverance, character; and character, hope. And hope does not disappoint us, because God has poured out his love into our hearts by the Holy Spirit, whom he has given us.

[34] Hoop vir depressielyers Page 14

[35] Ibid. Page 34

[36] Ibid. Page 15

[37] Treatment of depression – Page 18

[38] Ibid. Page 18 - 19

[39] Depression information for you – Pamphlet

[40] Hoop vir depressielyers – Page 50

[41] Treatment of depression Page 1

[42] We could now summarize it as follows: if my goal is to feel significant, and my basic assumption is that a lot of money will make me feel significant, I will devise a strategy of goal-oriented behaviour (how to make a lot of money) in order to reach that goal.

[43] Philippians 4:4

[44] Philippians 4:6

[45] Therapeutic Psychology – Page 417

[46] It is this we need to change: the basic assumptions about what we need in order to have our most basic needs met

[47] Note that her resentment is directed at her husband, so that he would normally also be the "external circumstance" to which the feeling is related.

[48] Counselors, comforters and friends – Pages 84 - 85

[49] Ibid. Page 86 - 87

[50] Ibid. Pages 89 - 90

[51] 2 Co 12:9

[52] Is 1:18

Don't miss out!

Visit the website below and you can sign up to receive emails whenever Carl Davis publishes a new book. There's no charge and no obligation.

https://books2read.com/r/B-A-ZAXZ-EECUC

BOOKS 2 READ

Connecting independent readers to independent writers.

Also by Carl Davis

Ek, is Dawid Soeker

A Brief History Of Christianity In Africa

Icing the Eskimo - The Art of Aggressive Sales

Introduction to Pastoral Counselling

Nuclear Faith

Toxic Pulpit

Van Paradegrond tot Pastorie

Group Dynamics and Motivation

Introduction to Leadership and Management

Pastoral counselling models for perinatal and postpartum episodes

Basic New Testament Survey

Help! I'm managing personnel

So......You want to be a Waiter

The Art of Preaching

Eternal Logos: The Evolution of Scriptural Interpretation: From Ancient Methodology to Postmodern Perspectives

Ewige Woord Die Evolusie van Skrifuitleg: Van Antieke Metodiek tot Postmoderne Perspektiewe

Teaching Ministry

The Funny Side Of Reasoning - Fallacies, principles and typologies in the modern business world.

Passion Unleashed: Igniting The Future With Purpose.

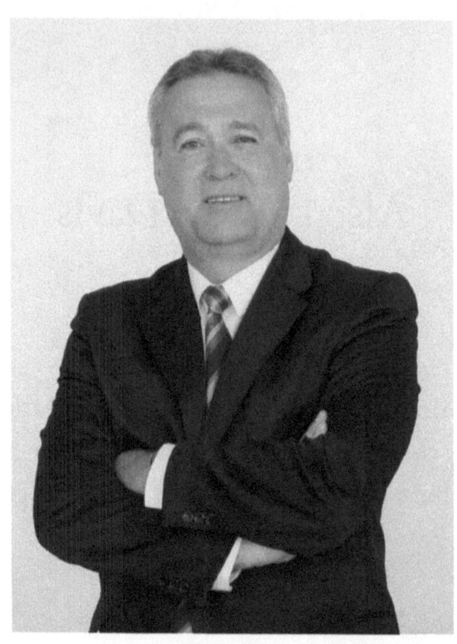

About the Author

Carl Davis holds a Doctorate in Missiology based upon research of Organizational Growth in the Post Modern Society.I started my work life serving in the South African Defence Force – first at the Recruiting Division, then moving to a Medical Command where I served as a Generalist Personnel Officer. For the last two years of my service, I was tasked with the Personnel management of the Integration process, inclusive of entrance and exit strategies.After honorable discharge after more than 10 years in the South African Defence Force, I took up the post of Managing Director of a Non-Government Organization, established to uplift impoverished communities in and around Potchefstroom, while also appointed as a part-time lecturer of undergraduates (specifically on leadership).Three years later I was appointed as Rector, managing an Educational Institute with 4000 students spread over 36 African countries. While in this position I had the opportunity to lecture extensively abroad and published various articles on leadership; with specific emphasis on motivation and group dynamics. I am a strong believer in utilizing a blended and integrated approach in all of the training (including the new material which I developed) I developed which included – Leadership (within a Faith based community), andragogy, and Cultural Diversity management.I am also a graduate of the University of Stellenbosch's Facilitative Leadership Programme (BUVTON), consulting and facilitating with organizations that are "stuck" (- Alice Mann 1998-) specifically in the process of change management.